AF570693

The Future of Pharmaceuticals

The Future of Pharmaceuticals

The Changing Environment for New Drugs

Clement Bezold, Ph.D.
Director
Institute for Alternative Futures
Washington, D.C.

Foreword by Alvin Toffler

A Wiley Medical Publication
John Wiley & Sons
New York Chichester Brisbane Toronto

Library of Congress Cataloging in Publication Data

Bezold, Clement.

The future of pharmaceuticals.

(A Wiley medical publication)

Includes index.

1. Pharmaceutical research. 2. Drug trade- - Technological innovations. 3. Pharmaceutical policy- - United States. I. Title.

RS122.B47 338.4'76151'072073 80-22603

ISBN 0-471-08343-7

Printed in the United States of America

10 9 8 7 6 5 4 3 2 1

Foreword

Although this book focuses on the future of the pharmaceutical industry, it has a second, hidden table of contents: it is also a book about the future of Congress.

In *The Third Wave* and elsewhere (including speeches given in the Congress) I have argued that today's rapid social and technological changes are making our political institutions obsolete. Designed for a late agrarian or early industrial age, the U.S. Congress today is overloaded with information, drenched and deluged with data it can neither digest properly nor apply intelligently.

And this is true not only of the Congress alone. The same can be said about the House of Commons, the Japanese Diet, the Supreme Soviet, and most other legislative bodies in the high technology world, all the way down to local town councils.

Because most of our legislative processes were designed for a slower moving, less complex world, lawmakers often pass sweeping legislation without examining their own subterranean assumptions and without systematically attempting to anticipate the long-range effects (especially the side effects) of their actions.

This book grows out of an attempt to improve the legislative process as it pertains to one fast-changing field, the future of pharmaceuticals. Regardless of how one feels about the substantive issues in this field—the rising cost of research and development, the slowdown in new drug introductions, the shift toward preventive medicine, the experiments with recombinant DNA—it is interesting for the light it casts on the legislative process.

Clement Bezold and the Institute for Alternative Futures have spent a great deal of time and effort in recent years studying and attempting to enhance legislative foresight. These are activities worthy of both intellectual and financial support.

ALVIN TOFFLER

Preface

Foresight is the term chosen to describe a variety of techniques that Congress and state and local legislatures use to identify emerging issues, to consider the long-term impacts of current decisions, and to relate multiple policies to long-term goals. As part of its work in the area of legislative foresight, the Institute for Alternative Futures designed a series of meetings called Foresight Seminars on Pharmaceutical Research and Development, conducted primarily for congressional staff and held on Capitol Hill. Topics for each of the six seminars that made up the first series, held during 1978 and 1979, combined current legislative concerns with forecasts for pharmaceutical R & D policy. They were chosen by the Institute in consultation with an informal advisory group consisting of congressional staff people and representatives from industry, academia, and public interest groups. Each of the seminars brought together three experts with divergent perspectives from the research community, industry, public interest groups, or government agencies. The papers prepared for these seminars and the highlights of the discussions provide the background for the six chapters of this book.

Throughout the series, forecasts were used to consider the future of pharmaceuticals. Chapter 1 reviews the potential breakthroughs that drug R & D might produce by the end of this century. Some of the forecasts developed in the late 1960s turn out to be overly optimistic, while significant breakthroughs appear likely in a variety of areas. The discussion considers the role of industry and of serendipity—the happy accidents—in drug discoveries. The impact of the current drug regulation system, put in place by the 1962 amendments to the Food, Drug, and Cosmetic Act of 1938, is reviewed along with the arguments about whether the amendments virtually bankrupted the drug R & D effort or whether they saved the industry.

Looking ahead in any policy area requires consideration of the assumptions underlying the current policies as well as the potential alternatives decisionmakers face. In the case of policy for pharmaceutical R & D, alternative approaches to health care, both through preventive strategies and therapeutic interventions, must be considered. Chapter 2 describes the rise in popularity of a host of alternatives to our conventional, largely allopathic, form of medicine. It sets out the historical and scientific background of medicine in the United States, including medicine's focus on suppression of symptoms and separation of the mind and body. It also looks at the regulatory system, particularly the scientific requirements for proving safety and efficacy that have evolved around the pharmaceutical component of medicine and the questions raised by the alternative approaches. As the discussion indicates, there is disagreement about the interpretation, much less the resolution, of these questions.

Chapter 3 returns to the mainstream of current thinking and examines the relationship between government regulation and the incentives for pharmaceutical firms to pursue the discovery and development of new drugs. The current cost for the average new drug is estimated to be $54 million—$30 million for research and $24 million for development. This includes the cost for the compounds that are considered but are not useful, as well as the company's return on investment. To recoup this investment, companies pursue commercially viable drugs, ones capable of generating at least $10 million in yearly global sales, as well as more attractive "jackpot" drugs whose yearly sales exceed $100 million. The cost for drug R & D increased sixfold from the 1950s through the early 1970s. One-third of the increased cost appears to have been the result of more stringent requirements on the part of the Food and Drug Administration (FDA) in implementing the 1962 amendments. Divergent opinions on the impact of the Drug Regulation Reform Act of 1979 are reviewed, as are the options it gives the FDA for more flexibility in its decision-making.

Chapter 4 considers the potential impact of National Health Insurance on pharmaceutical R & D. Since there is no clear-cut answer and little research on this issue, the chapter outlines the various links in the chain from increased physician visits and physician prescribing behavior through the sales, profit, R & D budgets, and research targeting of pharmaceutical firms. The discussion section reviews the forecasts and insights generated by seminar participants. A chapter appendix by Dr. Michael Riddiough, senior analyst at the Congressional Office of Technology Assessment, presents a more detailed consideration of the potential impact of National Health Insurance on new drugs.

The Drug Regulation Reform Act of 1979 proposed the establishment of a National Center for Drug Science to focus attention on research for drug breakthroughs, particularly on "orphan" drugs, those of limited commercial value, and on policy questions, such as how safety and efficacy requirements should relate to changing perceptions of biological science and drug usage. Chapter 5 presents arguments for and against the establishment of the center as well as some of its potential impacts.

Chapter 6 considers the role of recombinant DNA techniques in pharmaceutical R & D. Recombinant DNA techniques are on the verge of revolutionizing important aspects of the pharmaceutical field, both because of their capacity to produce biologically active proteins such as insulin and interferon and because of the possibility that certain diseases, such as sickle cell anemia, could be eliminated through gene replacement therapy. The recent developments in Congress and in research and industrial laboratories are reviewed, and the potential ethical problems this technology poses are examined.

Together, these chapters and the insights they generated represent a major step toward the systematic examination of the future of pharmaceutical R & D. They were designed to broaden the framework and lengthen the time horizon within which such issues are usually examined and to raise questions about the implicit assumptions that underlie policymaking in this area. They deliberately sought to stimulate controversy and to facilitate insights on the discovery, use, and regulation of new pharmaceutical products.

CLEMENT BEZOLD

Acknowledgments

The credit for this book rests in a variety of places; the blame for its shortcomings rests with me. The book is the product of an intellectual exercise—aiding congressional staff and a community of others active in the area of pharmaceutical R & D to look ahead more systematically. The first credit goes to the participants, both on and off Capitol Hill, in the Foresight Seminars on Pharmaceutical Research and Development and to the 18 speakers who enlivened the six seminars.

Designing the series so that it focused on the future but had enough consideration of present concerns to be relevant to the day-to-day work of congressional staffpeople was greatly aided by a core of advisers, among whom I would particularly like to thank Janice Zarro, Michael Riddiough, and Alan Fox. In addition I appreciate the assistance of Peter Goldschmidt, Stanley Molner, Hadassah Tucker, James Turner, and Erol Caglarcan.

The seminars were made possible by a grant from Hoffmann-La Roche Inc. I would particularly like to acknowledge the risk that Hoffmann-La Roche was willing to undertake in supporting an open, experimental educational series over which I had full editorial control, as well as the enthusiastic support of John H. Wood, former director of public affairs.

Finally, I would like to express my gratitude to my colleague and sometime editor, Rosemarie Philips, my wife, for her assistance throughout the Foresight Seminars.

CLEMENT BEZOLD

Contents

The Future of Pharmaceuticals

1

The Future of Pharmaceuticals: Breakthrough Possibilities, Development Constraints, and Policy Questions

In *Who Shall Live?: Health, Economics and Social Choice*, Victor Fuchs noted that drugs are the key to modern medicine. "Six dollars are spent on hospitals and physicians for every dollar spent on drugs, but without drugs the effectiveness of hospitals and physicians would be enormously diminished." The great power of drugs has developed during the last 40 years—decades referred to as the atomic, electronic, and space ages. But as Fuchs pointed out, "measured by impact on people's lives [these years] might just as well be called the 'drug age.' "[1]

What is the future of new pharmaceutical therapies in this era? What will biomedical and related drug research and development yield between now and the end of this century?

During this age of new pharmaceutical therapies, medical care has advanced beyond mere diagnosis of certain diseases. With drugs and vaccines, medical science is able to reduce the incidence of infectious diseases such as pneumonia, tuberculosis, typhoid, whooping cough, poliomyelitis, measles, diphtheria, and tetanus; smallpox has been eradicated through an aggressive vaccination program. Many of these advances began in the 1930s and 1940s with the development of sulfa drugs and antibiotics. More recently, a variety of drugs have been developed that have been used with great success to treat arthritis, high blood pressure, psychoneurotic conditions, diabetes, epilepsy, circulatory diseases, and certain bacterial infections.

[1]Victor Fuchs, *Who Shall Live?: Health, Economics and Social Choice* (New York: Basic Books, 1974), p. 106.

Drug research involves a variety of approaches to the identification, invention, and discovery of a potential new therapy:

- empirical screening of large numbers of chemical compounds thought to have therapeutic capabilities
- molecular modification of existing therapies in order to reduce side effects or improve efficacy
- basic research into chemical and biomedical areas such as cellular biology and molecular structure
- investigations of foreign chemicals that lead to the discovery of entirely new therapeutic properties of the molecule

Such approaches to drug discovery are either planned or deliberate. Serendipity—the unexpected finding in the clinic or laboratory of the potential utility of a compound—is believed to account for up to 50% of all major scientific breakthroughs.

Drug development begins with a decision to make the drug available for human use and ends when the first quantities are marketed. Although the research process takes place in industry laboratories, government research institutes, universities, and other nonprofit organizations and laboratories, the development process is performed almost exclusively by drug companies.

In the United States the development process is regulated by the 1938 Food, Drug, and Cosmetic Act, particularly its 1962 amendments (see Chapters 2 & 3). When a compound is chosen for development, initial screening in rodents and other animals follows. Specialists from numerous disciplines become involved, and developmental chemists undertake large-scale synthesis of the compound. If continued testing suggests a significant therapeutic effect, toxicity studies are initiated. Generally, the drug is administered to dogs or monkeys in the dosage form proposed for human use (though usually at a higher dose-unit-per body weight for the animals than for expected human use), and careful research is done to determine any toxic effects. If tests to this point suggest that the drug is safe and effective, physician researchers begin carefully controlled testing in human volunteers. Approval of the Food and Drug Administration (FDA) to market the drug is granted only after satisfactory clinical trials and may include a requirement for postmarketing surveillance of the drug and its potential side effects (see Figure 1-1 in discussion highlights of this chapter and Chapter 3).

The effectiveness of this approach to drug development is the focus of active debate. There is agreement, however, that drug companies are virtually the only entities with the extensive resources needed to develop and market a new drug.

FORECASTING THE FUTURE

What social benefits can be expected from drug research in the next 20 or more years? During the last 15 years, forecasting has become more systematic; a number of studies on drugs have appeared that can suggest an answer. These studies generally begin with a disclaimer, since accurate forecasting is virtually impossible. Some investigators search for a particular finding to be confirmed through systematic research, while others may serendipitously stumble onto breakthroughs. Thus, drug forecasts can provide a context for thinking about policy options, but they cannot predict precisely which new drugs will be available. Nor can forecasts answer questions that policymakers must face regarding relative effectiveness of drug therapy compared to other forms of disease prevention and treatment.

SCENARIOS FOR PHARMACEUTICALS

Most forecasts in the area of drug development—and all those reported below—were generated by expert opinion. In one popular forecasting technique, the Delphi survey, a panel of experts is polled in two or more rounds, during which they adjust their forecasts in light of the collective response on the previous round. One of the first major Delphi surveys of the pharmaceutical industry was conducted in 1968 by Dr. A. Douglas Bender for SmithKline and French Laboratories.[2] Thirty-five experts expressed their opinions on future developments in health care, therapy, biomedical research, and medical education. A more recent survey of the future of the medical field was taken in 1976 by *Medical World News*.[3] A modified Delphi poll was used to survey 23 leading experts in various medical specialties on the clinical advances most likely to become conventional medical practice, assuming current levels of support for medical research.

The SmithKline and French survey and the *Medical World News* survey indicated a number of developments that would take place by the years 1980, 1990, and 2000.

[2] A. Douglas Bender *et al.*, "Delphi Study Examines Developments in Medicine," *Futures*, Vol. 1, No. 4 (June, 1969), p. 289.

[3] David E. Leff, "Medicine 2000," *Medical World News* (January 24, 1977), pp. 44–54.

The year 1980[4,5]

- the therapeutic armamentarium of a first-term student in medical school in 1980 includes drugs for the cure or prevention of hypertension, edema, skeletal muscle spasm, autoimmune disease, fungal infections, drug dependence, thrombosis, obesity, anxiety, tension, depression, asthma, and dental caries; cell-specific therapy for certain neoplasms, a hepatitis vaccine, nonnutrient foods for obesity control, and a variety of special diets for patients with such diseases as atherosclerosis and phenylketonuria will also be available; drugs and other new methods controlling male and female fertility will be at the physician's disposal
- negligible morbidity and mortality for childhood malignancies, notably leukemia and Hodgkin's disease, as a result of new therapeutic regimens
- highly accurate enzyme and radioimmunoassay screening of persons with a high risk of cancer
- H2 blockers for routine treatment of ulcers and erosive hyperacidity
- H2 receptor-blocking agents for treating peptic ulcers are in their fourth year of clinical trial
- satisfactory clinical management of essential hypertension
- successful treatment of herpes simplex
- medical treatment of schizophrenia, depression, and other mental disorders
- effective monitoring of drug therapy
- nonaddictive analgesia for intractable pain

The year 1990

- therapeutic regimens for all pediatric cancers
- complete detectability of cancer through enzymes and radioimmunoassay
- chemotherapy or immunotherapy for gastrointestinal malignancies as well as kidney, bladder, and prostate cancers
- dramatic reduction in the incidence of sudden cardiac death and myocardial damage from severe obstructionary coronary artery disease
- vaccine to prevent diabetes
- treatment of psoriasis and melanoma

[4]Bender *et al.*, *op. cit.*, p. 289.

[5]Leff, *op. cit.*, pp. 44–54. Last nine items of list reprinted from *Medical World News*, copyright © 1977, McGraw-Hill, Inc.

- prevention of all important viral diseases by immunization with purified antigens
- manipulation of cellular immune reactions in delayed hypersensitivity, autoimmune disease, suppression of fertility, and organ transplantation

The year 2000

- prevention of heritable diseases
- prevention of mental illness, nephritis, degenerative vascular disease, arthritis, and, increasingly, cancer
- nontoxic and almost completely effective cancer chemotherapy
- treatment of psychiatric disorders by correction of molecular basis of pathogenesis

FORECASTS FOR BIOMEDICAL RESEARCH

Another approach to forecasting is to identify key individuals who can relate forecasts to underlying causes, or in this case, the research areas that will ultimately have the highest payoff for pharmaceutical treatment of disease. Lewis Thomas, president of the Memorial Sloan Kettering Cancer Center and author of *Lives of a Cell*,[6] and Max Tishler, university professor of science at Wesleyan University and former president of Merck, Sharp & Dohme Laboratories, are prominent experts who have provided their own forecasts.

Lewis Thomas, writing in 1977, stated that "the major diseases of human beings have become approachable biological puzzles, ultimately solvable. It follows from this that it is now possible to begin thinking about a human society relatively free of disease."[7] Thomas felt that the experience of the past 50 years suggests two principles about human disease. First, it is necessary to know a great deal about underlying mechanisms before one can really act effectively. Second, for every disease there is a single key mechanism that dominates all others. For example, he proposed that while dozens of separate influences, including environmental carcinogens and many sorts of virus, launch cancer, there is a single switch at the center of things. Schizophrenia will turn out to be a neurochemical disorder in which some single central chemical event has gone wrong. Rheumatoid

[6]Lewis Thomas, *Lives of a Cell: Notes of a Biology Watcher* (New York: Bantam Books, 1974).

[7]Lewis Thomas, "Biomedical Science and Human Health: The Long-range Prospect," *Daedalus* (Summer, 1977), p. 168.

arthritis, coronary occlusion, and stroke will all be found to have single key mechanisms. According to Thomas, many of these mechanisms may involve a common set of problems now being addressed by many researchers: How do cells and tissues become labeled for what they are, what are the forces that govern the orderly development and differentiation of tissues and organs, and how do errors in the process occur?

Over a decade ago, Max Tishler, writing with Robert Denkewalter, forecast that great strides would be made in treating infectious diseases. He predicted vaccines for rubella, mumps, and viral hepatitis, and more effective drugs against malaria, schistosomiasis, amebiasis, and trypanosomiasis. Better drugs, though less significant advances, would come in the areas of hypertension, mental health, metabolic disorders, and cancer treatments. Yet Tishler felt that significant breakthroughs in solving the problems of atherosclerosis, genetic diseases, schizophrenia, osteoporosis, and cancer would have to await a deeper understanding of biochemical processes.[8]

Tishler and Thomas agree that the most promising areas for fundamental research breakthroughs are the fields of neurobiology, immunology, molecular biology, cellular differentiation, cell membrane studies, and genetics.

There is disagreement in the research community over the appropriate balance between basic and applied research and the relative distribution across specialties. There is also less optimism on the part of some clinical researchers and those involved in moving drugs through the approval process. But, by and large, there is agreement on our ultimate ability to control most diseases.

[8]Robert G. Denkewalter and Max Tishler, "Drug Research—Whence and Whither," *Progress in Drug Research*, ed. Ernest Jucker (Basel, Switzerland: Birkhauser, 1966).

HIGHLIGHTS OF THE DISCUSSION

In trying to assess the future of the pharmaceutical industry, consideration must be given to the question of whether, as some have charged, the industry is in its death throes. There are those who feel that the industry's problems are the result of costly government regulations, while others believe that the industry's diminishing role results from a combination of its own failure to do the rigorous research necessary to identify and mitigate the side effects of drugs and of popular neglect as more consumers reject drugs in favor of other therapies.

According to Frank Standaert, chairman of the Department of Pharmacology at Georgetown University Schools of Medicine and Dentistry, drugs will continue to be the most important form of therapy prescribed by physicians for two major reasons: drugs are usually more economical than other treatments, and drugs are the most practical means of therapy for large numbers of patients. He noted, however, that for all its successes in the recent past, pharmacology is still a new science, and drug therapy is complicated, potentially dangerous, and inadequately understood.

In reviewing the forecasts, Standaert agreed that drugs will bring about a range of improved health conditions during the next 20 years but cautioned that these improvements will take longer than originally estimated, particularly for those drugs for which forecasts were developed in 1968. In comparing the 1968 and 1976 forecasts for drug breakthroughs, he noted a difference in the level of optimism and fundamental changes in thinking that occurred between the earlier and later period:

> The need to understand the basic biological and pharmacologic interactions as a requisite for more effective pharmaceutical therapies is now better recognized. Earlier drug breakthroughs exhausted our available knowledge, and the advance of our understanding in some areas has been slower than was anticipated in 1968. Ironically, in 1978—as a result of increased knowledge—some diseases appear less curable than they had 10 years ago.
>
> Certain diseases such as drug dependence are increasingly seen as problems requiring behavioral rather than pharmaceutical therapies. More attention has been focused on drugs as part of the problem rather than

part of the solution to health problems such as anxiety, tension, and depression.

Standaert felt that some of the 1968 forecasts were accurate, or nearly accurate, some were only partially correct, but that many must still await further research. For example, the forecast for 1980 accurately predicted that H2 blockers would be used routinely for the treatment of ulcers and erosive hyperacidity and that H2 receptor-blocking agents for treatment of peptic ulcers would undergo clinical trials. The forecasts for clinical management of essential hypertension and treatment of schizophrenia, depression, and other mental disorders were, however, only partially correct. The management of hypertension with drugs has improved because better understanding of the pharmokinetics of hypertension permits better management with existing drugs. On the other hand, few significant new compounds have been introduced for the nonaddictive treatment of intractable pain, nor has effective monitoring of drug therapy become a widespread practice.

Standaert predicted that during the next 10 to 25 years, drug therapies will be developed to prevent or cure hypertension, severe skeletal muscle spasms, autoimmune disease, asthma, and thrombosis. He further claimed that drug therapies for the prevention or cure of edema, although a condition secondary to heart or kidney disease, will be developed. He was less confident that cell-specific therapies for neoplasms or drugs to prevent dental caries will be developed or that improvements in drug regimes—the ways particular drugs are used—will yield significant therapeutic gain.

Using a flow chart (Figure 1-1), Standaert pointed out the increasing cost and time required for the development process due to the need to protect human subjects, ethical dilemmas facing those running clinical trials, and rising hospital costs.

Jerome Schnee, a leading academic economist in the pharmaceutical area, added to and expanded on Standaert's list of problems affecting the development process. He felt that drug development regulations established in 1962 have had a major influence on industry trends.

First, there has been a decline in the number of new chemical entities introduced each year. Before 1962 the average was 50 to 60 per year. Since 1962, however, the average has dropped to only 17 per year. This drop includes all chemical entities, not just those that are considered to be of particular medical importance.

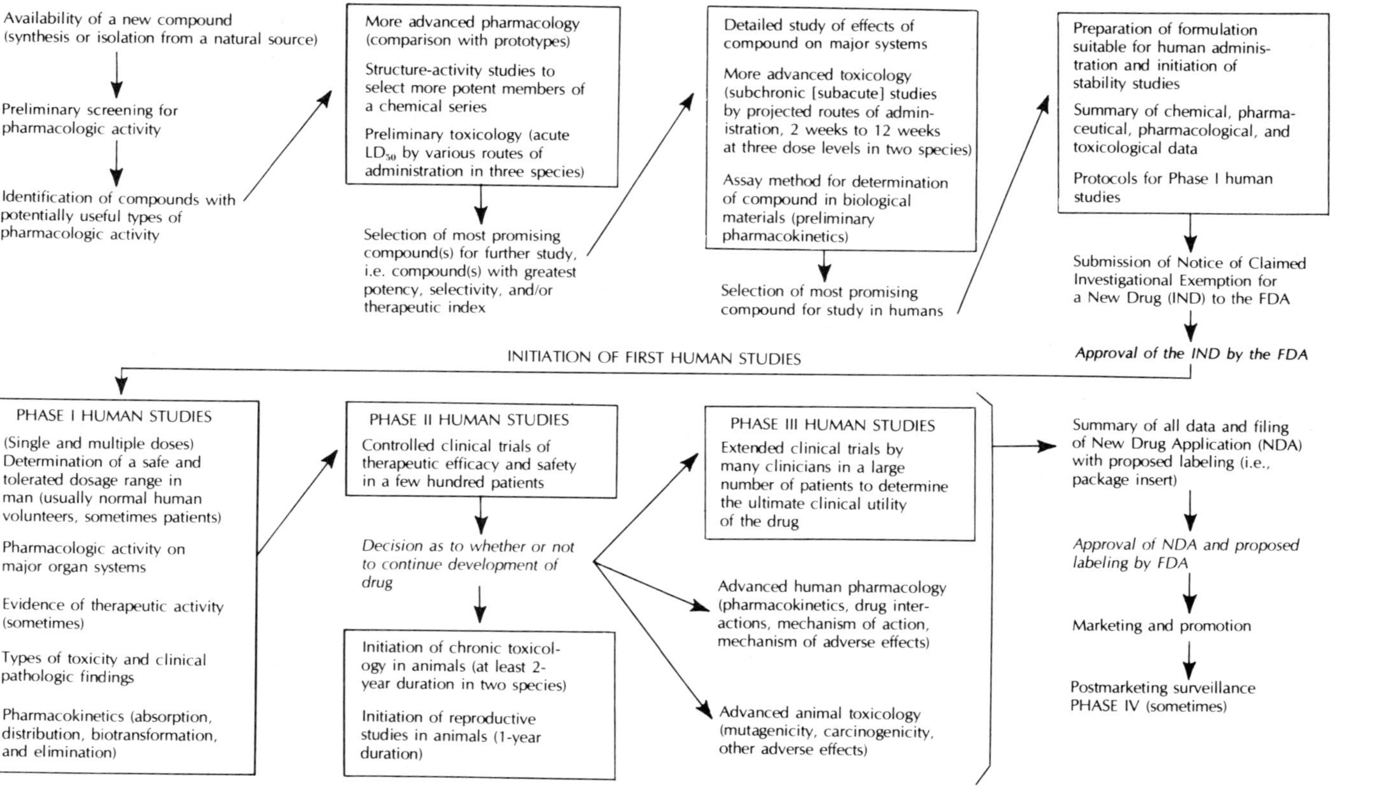

Figure 1-1. New drug development. [SOURCE: Frank G. Standaert, Department of Pharmacology, Georgetown University Schools of Medicine and Dentistry, Washington, D.C.]

Second, the cost in dollars and time of developing a drug has risen from an average of $1 million and 2 years to $25 million and 7 to 10 years in the post-1962 environment. To illustrate this point, the director of research for a large pharmaceutical company explained that the figures for a particular recent budgeting put the company's costs at $15 million not including other operating (nonresearch) company expenses or an additional percentage computed for rate of return. This figure also does not include the costs of exploring drug possibilities that are subsequently rejected. Current estimates are that only 1 out of 10 compounds that begin the development process ever make it to the market. According to two recent studies, increased costs and time of development have resulted in a drop in return on research and development (R & D) investments to below 5%.

Third, there has been a movement of R & D resources out of the country—from 7% to 8% of companies' R & D budgets in the early 1960s to about 16% of current industry R & D.

Fourth, as smaller companies are less able to afford R & D, innovation has become concentrated in the larger firms, and even large companies have had to limit the number of potential innovations they pursue, thus reinforcing the concentration within therapeutic lines.

The most significant effect of these trends on the future availability of new drugs will be the reduction in corporate research efforts, including theory-based or basic research. During the 1970s about 90% of new chemical entities were discovered or originated in industry laboratories, but Schnee predicted that this output will drop and that drug firms will look increasingly to U.S. government and university research as well as to foreign companies for new drugs rather than discover them on their own. In addition, as one researcher pointed out, since in many cases serendipitous work—"happy accidents"—precipitated innovations, cutbacks in R & D will also lessen the chances for surprise leads.

James Turner, a public interest attorney and consumer advocate, characterized the pharmaceutical industry as dying, despite the fact that there is a legitimate need for pharmaceutical products, but he disagreed with Schnee's analysis of the effects of the 1962 regulations as the cause.

Turner argued that 1962 is an unrealistic date to select as the beginning point for looking at the decline in introduction of new pharmaceutical products. He claimed that introduction of new chemical entities actually peaked before 1959 and that the decline in the rate of introduction was heightened in that and subsequent years by the thalidomide crisis (see Figures 3-3 and 3-4). As a result, public confidence in pharmaceuticals plummeted, and the situation was aggravated by a major conflict-of-interest scandal in the FDA.

The 1962 amendments, according to Turner, actually represented a government seal of approval, an assurance to the public of a minimum confidence level, that allowed the industry to continue to function. Turner claimed that without the 1962 amendments, there would be no pharmaceutical industry at all in the United States today.

As for the flight of R & D funds overseas, Turner suggested that although the problem may be related in part to regulatory costs, it more likely reflects the general trend toward multinational corporate activity that would have affected pharmaceutical research at this time anyway.

Turner explained the decline in the pharmaceutical industry not as a result not of government regulations but of the public "voting with its feet" for a growing range of alternatives to drug therapies such as nutritional therapy, chiropractic, and even homeopathy, which have fewer negative side effects. He highlighted three areas—vaccines, birth control pills, and oral drugs for diabetes—in which negative side effects of pharmaceuticals could have been targeted much more explicitly. These effects could then have been eliminated or those people in danger of suffering from them could have been properly warned at the beginning of treatment. The Salk polio vaccine, for example, paralyzed monkeys in 1957 premarketing tests. This effect was ignored until some 200 to 250 people contracted polio from the vaccine. Use of the drug was then temporarily prohibited, and within 30 days the problem was solved and the drug was again offered to the public. Turner suggested that if drug companies would work to identify the characteristics of people likely to experience negative side effects, drug therapies would be more helpful from the outset.

2

Alternatives to Drug Therapy: Implications for Pharmaceutical R & D

". . . The assumptions that underlie a research project are far more interesting and far more important than anything actually done in research itself."

Norbert Weiner

The role of the federal government with regard to pharmaceutical therapies is twofold: (1) to promote the discovery and development of new and effective pharmaceutical therapies and (2) to regulate, on the bases of safety and efficacy, the general availability of such therapies in the marketplace.

This chapter will analyze the contexts in which health care choices are made. It will examine the growing popularity and acceptance of a variety of alternative therapies and the issues that their increasing availability raises for government policymakers in the area of pharmaceuticals. In the process, this discussion will examine the assumptions underlying both pharmaceutical therapies and alternative approaches to health care.

IMPORTANCE OF CLARIFYING ASSUMPTIONS

Because policy decisions that shape legislation are often made in response to specific historical circumstances, they are often based, either explicitly or implicitly, on narrow assumptions. These assumptions are seldom examined thoroughly. Moreover, subsequent debate on amendments to legislation often fails to reconsider the original assumptions in light of experience. For example, the Hill-Burton Act of 1954 was passed to meet a need for more hospitals. The assumption that more hospitals were needed was not questioned until after the Act had contributed to the overbuilding of hospitals.

In the area of pharmaceutical policy, it is generally assumed that new drug discovery is a good thing, particularly if the drug represents a significant therapeutic gain. Yet, as patients and health care providers are presented with a more diversified choice of therapies, it is appropriate to question whether treatment with prescription drugs is more desirable than other available therapies and whether policymakers should direct more effort toward preventative or health promoting strategies than discovering new treatments.

The rise of alternative therapies suggests that if comparative efficacy is to be the standard by which the FDA decides which therapies will be available to the consumer, a broader definition of comparative efficacy may be needed. Alternatively, if the market mechanism is to be the arbiter of comparative efficacy, then regulatory policy might act to overcome current market imperfections by making it easier for safe, new drugs to reach the market. Specifically, regulators and policymakers may act to deal with (1) the absence of effective reporting systems on the efficacy of drugs and other therapies in use, (2) the absence of a reliable nongovernmental entity to report results of efficacy tests and make recommendations, (3) ineffectual patient/consumer education programs, and (4) an educational system for health providers that favors conventional treatment modalities over health promotion and over treatment by nontraditional modalities. (Appendix A, page 27, identifies a variety of policy options in these areas.)

HISTORY OF GOVERNMENT REGULATION OF DRUGS

Although drugs have been an important form of therapy for centuries, the past four decades have witnessed the most significant progress in pharmaceutical R & D in history. Despite the fact that drugs have been invaluable in alleviating suffering and curing disease, they have also been used fraudulently.[1] Public dissatisfaction with widespread deception in food and drug claims led to the passage of the Pure Food and Drug Act of 1906. The law dealt primarily with food and had little impact on impure or unsafe drugs.

[1]James Harvey Young, *The Toadstool Millionaires* (Princeton, N.J.: Princeton University Press, 1971, and *The Medical Messiahs* (Princeton, N.J.: Princeton University Press, 1967).

Since 1906 the federal government has acted twice to increase the stringency of regulations governing the marketing of new drugs. In both cases, passage of proposals for increased regulation followed widely publicized tragedies involving the use of insufficiently tested, unsafe drugs.

The Food, Drug, and Cosmetic Act was passed in 1938, shortly after the death of more than 100 people who had taken "elixir sulfanilamide," a potent antibacterial agent containing the poisonous solvent diethylene glycol (an ingredient in antifreeze). This law instituted the "safety" standard still followed today: it ruled that no new product could be marketed until the manufacturer presented convincing evidence of the drug's safety to the FDA. The law also stiffened regulations against false and misleading advertising, required warning labels, banned dangerous drugs, strengthened enforcement procedures, and made penalties for violations more severe.

Nearly 25 years later in 1962, the 1938 law was changed as a result of hearings begun in 1959 by Senator Estes Kefauver. Senator Kefauver's hearings were prompted by his concern that existing regulations permitted the introduction of new drugs of questionable efficacy. He felt that this resulted from a combination of patent protection of new chemical entities, consumer and physician ignorance, and minimal incentives for physicians to consider the costs to patients of prescription drugs.[2] However, the thalidomide episode—the birth in 1962 and 1963 of deformed children to mothers who had taken the drug during pregnancy—is often cited as the impetus for amendments to the 1938 Food, Drug, and Cosmetics Act.[3]

The 1962 amendments had two major objectives: (1) closer federal control of premarket testing of new drugs and (2) altered criteria for marketing approval of new drugs. They empowered the FDA to require companies to submit a satisfactory investigational new drug (IND) form before it granted permission to conduct clinical testing in humans. An IND must contain comprehensive data gathered from extensive preclinical safety and efficacy testing in animals. Also, the 1962 amendments:

> . . . added a proof-of-efficacy requirement to the proof-of-safety requirement of the 1938 law. No new drug may now be marketed unless

[2]Jerome Schnee, "Government Control of Therapeutic Drugs: Impact and Issues," *The Pharmaceutical Industry*, ed. Cotton M. Lindsay (New York: John Wiley & Sons, 1978), pp. 10–11.

[3]Milton Silverman and Philip R. Lee, *Pills, Profits and Politics* (Berkeley: University of California Press, 1974), p. 96.

> and until the FDA determines not only that the drug is safe, as required under the 1938 law, but also that there is "substantial evidence," according to statutory scientific criteria, that it is effective for its intended use. An effective drug, in this context, is one which the FDA determines, on the basis of adequate clinical studies, will meet the claims made for it by the manufacturer. Further, promotion of all prescription drugs can claim no more than the effects established before the FDA and must include a summary of the side effects, contraindications, and effectiveness.[4]

Intense legislation activity provoked by crisis is seldom accompanied by thorough fundamental analysis of assumptions. Thus, while significant changes were made in 1938 and 1962, there was no attempt to examine assumptions underlying drug therapy. The noncrisis atmosphere surrounding current consideration of the Drug Regulatory Reform Act and the rising holistic health movement provide an opportunity to study the assumptions behind various modes of health care.

CONTRIBUTIONS OF DRUGS TO HEALTH

Victor Fuchs has written, "drugs are the key of modern medicine. Surgery, radiotherapy, and diagnostic tests are all important, but the ability of health care providers to alter health outcomes . . . depends primarily on drugs." He points out that the ability of medical science to cure or prevent disease has advanced significantly in recent decades.

> [By 1925] some advances had been made in surgery, but the death rates from tuberculosis, influenza and pneumonia, and other infectious diseases were still extremely high. With the introduction and wide use of sulfonamide and penicillin, however, the death rate in the United States from influenza and pneumonia fell by more than 8% annually from 1935 to 1950. (The annual rate of decline from 1900 and 1935 had been only 2%.) In the case of tuberculosis, while some progress had been made since the turn of the century, the rate of decline in the death rate accelerated appreciably after the adoption of penicillin, streptomycin, and PAS (paraaminosalicylic acid) in the late 1940s and of isoniazid in the early 1950s. New drugs and vaccines developed since the 1920s have also been strikingly effective against typhoid, whooping cough, poliomyelitis, measles, diphtheria, and tetanus; more recently great

[4]Schnee, *op. cit.*, p. 12.

advances have been made in hormonal drugs, antihypertension drugs, antihistamines, anticoagulants, antipsychotic drugs, and antidepressants.[5]

The economic impact of these drugs in terms of reducing the cost of illness amounts to billions of dollars per year. Savings are brought about by reducing the need to treat, hospitalize, and provide long-term care for victims of disease. For example, introduction of antituberculosis drugs reduced hospital costs by $4 billion during the period from 1954 to 1969. Measles vaccine averted millions of cases of measles and thousands of incidences of fetal complications resulting in mental retardation, thus saving about $180 million yearly.[6]

QUESTIONING OF CONVENTIONAL MEDICINE

In 1977 the number of patient visits to physicians fell by 11% from the previous year. In part this reduction reflects a growing disillusionment with conventional medicine despite its many accomplishments. Of the increasing number of criticisms of traditional medicine, the most well known are Ivan Illich's discussion of iatrogenic (physician-induced) diseases and Rick Carlson's analysis of the "end of medicine."[7] However, the most prevalent criticisms of conventional medicine accompanying the rise of new health alternatives are those based on research in the fields of ecology and nutrition.

The Ecological Critique

According to proponents of the ecological critique of conventional medicine, current medical practices largely ignore the environmental causes of disease. John Powles's analysis is typical.

> Industrial man throws his energies into the technical mastery of nature by working on numerous independent fronts. In medicine, he has interposed a complex technology between himself and disease. This technology is mostly of an engineering character, that is, designed to repair disordered systems within sick individuals. Yet, the evidence suggests

[5] Victor Fuchs, *Who Shall Live?: Health, Economics and Social Choice* (New York: Basic Books, 1974), p. 106.

[6] Silverman and Lee, *op. cit.*, p. 14.

[7] Ivan Illich, *Medical Nemesis: The Expropriation of Health* (New York: Bantam Books, 1976); Rick J. Carlson, *The End of Medicine* (New York: John Wiley & Sons, 1976).

> that he owes his standard of health, not so much to the achievements of this technology as to the favorable nature of his new relationship with his environment with respect to his vulnerability to infections. Unfortunately, this new set of environmental relationships are unfavorable with respect to another cluster of diseases—diseases of adaptation such as arteriosclerosis, diabetes, hypertension, some forms of cancer, and accidents. Further, there is considerable evidence to suggest that improvements in the effectiveness of engineering medical technology (including drugs) are, when taken over all, only just managing to neutralize the increasing impact of diseases of maladaptation.[8]

Powles's study focused on Great Britain; however, similar American studies show that while private and public expenditures for health care have risen drastically, declining death rates from contagious diseases have been balanced by increased death rates from chronic and degenerative diseases. It has been suggested that, whereas modern medicine may provide symptomatic relief for certain diseases, it cannot control the basic healthiness or unhealthiness of our lifestyle, which is the basis of all disease.[9] In fact, a 20-year American study suggested that the socioeconomic composition of the population was a more important factor in explaining health status than increased health care resources.[10]

According to Victor Fuchs, the contribution of medical care to life expectancy in developed countries is very small. He notes that current medical knowledge cannot solve the problems of heart disease, cancer, accidents, emotional illness, and viral infections as effectively as the problems of infectious diseases were solved between 1930 and 1955. He recognizes, however, that "medical care performs other functions besides reducing mortality and morbidity. Particularly important are the caring functions (providing sympathy, reassurance, relief of anxiety), and the validation function (providing professional information about health status)."[11] The ecological critique deemphasizes medical science and charges that because of its technical, after-the-fact approach, the medical care system distracts individuals and societies from searching for the underlying causes of illness and from seeking preventative or promotive strategies.

[8]John Powles, "The Medicine of Industrial Man," *Ecologist*, Vol. 2 (1972), pp. 24ff.

[9]"The Point of Diminishing Returns," *East-West Journal* (October, 1978), p. 29.

[10]Michael K. Miller and C. Shannon Stokes, "Health Status, Health Resources, and Consolidated Structural Parameters: Implications for Public Health Care Policy," *Journal of Health and Social Behavior*, Vol. 19 (September, 1978), pp. 263–279.

[11]Fuchs, *op. cit.*, p. 144.

The Nutrition-Based Critique

Another assault on traditional medical thinking stems from extensive analysis of our nutritional practices and of the potential for nutritional therapies. In the 1970s, the Standard American Diet (SAD) included 250 pounds of meat, 130 pounds of refined and processed sugars, 295 12-ounce cans of soda per year, and a large percentage of highly refined carbohydrates and fast foods. Only 20% of calories came from fresh fruits, vegetables, and whole grains, whereas 40% of calories were derived from these sources in 1900. Epidemiological studies comparing diet and disease profiles of various groups link the SAD to the same diseases—heart disease, hypertension, diabetes, and cancer of the breast, stomach, and colon—identified by the ecological critique as resulting from industrialization.[12] While the relative effects of nutritional habits and industrialization have not been sorted out, both critiques implicitly question the value of drugs in developing long-term strategies for dealing with disease. Both suggest the importance of preventative, in contrast to therapeutic, approaches to health care.

Similar conclusions on the importance of nutrition for health were reached by the Senate Nutrition Committee chaired by Senator George McGovern. They were released along with a recommended personal nutrition policy in *Dietary Goals for the United States* and updated in 1977.

The Holistic Health Movement

The growing holistic health movement, which is based on the value of preventative or promotive health care, raises major questions about the assumptions underlying conventional medicine including drug therapy. The movement is made up of supporters of a multitude of health modalities, many of which have long histories and extensive use in practice. Some emphasize the social context of an individual's illness, while others emphasize the holism of the individual and regard personal growth exercises as an important component of active health promotion. Although there is some quackery and outright fraud within the holistic health movement, taken as a whole, it represents a growing popular challenge to established health policies and practices.

[12]Sam Keen, "The Pure, the Impure, and the Paranoid," *Psychology Today* (October, 1978), pp. 67–68, 73–79, 82, 87.

Modalities of the holistic health model share opposition to the conventional, or allopathic, medical model. Allopathy is treatment of disease with remedies that produce effects different from or opposite to those produced by the disease; for example, a patient with a fever would be given medication to lower body temperature. Traditional allopathic practice is reductionist: it assumes that the body and mind are separate entities that may be treated separately. In addition, the allopathic approach to health care is based on other implicit assumptions about the doctor-patient relationship, the role of the mind in illness, and the need for therapeutic intervention (see Table 2-1). The allopathic medical model defines illness and health at the microbiological level and assumes that the cause of illness lies within an individual. Society has little to do with the occurrence of illness. The course of therapy does not attempt to deal with the ill effects, if any, of an individual's environment. It is important to remember that the same assumptions underlying the allopathic medical model also underlie current federal policy in promoting and regulating the health care system. In contrast, the holistic health movement stresses the necessity of restructuring the social environment in order to achieve and maintain health effectively (see Figure 2-1). According to Hayes-Bautista and Harveston, ". . . both the individual and society are fit patients for the ministrations of holistic health care. Together, the ill individual and society are made healthy and positive actions are taken later to maintain that health level."[13] This approach to health includes family and work group therapy as well as measures aimed at identifying and eliminating environmental and social causes of illness.

An even larger segment of those involved in the holistic health movement support the concept of the holism of the person. Their concern for the unity of body and mind reflects one of the fundamental assumptions underlying the conventional medical model within which drug therapy is used. Jerome D. Frank, professor emeritus of medicine at Johns Hopkins University, has noted the following:

> Traditional Western medicine has been dominated by a viewpoint that dates back to the 17th century French philosopher-scientist Renè Descartes. It was Descartes who preached a division between mind and matter, with the human body being a form of matter. The medical

[13]David Hayes-Bautista and Dominic S. Harveston, "Holistic Health Care, *Social Policy* (March/April, 1977), p. 10.

Table 2-1. Assumptions Underlying Different Medical Models

Assumptions of the Allopathic Model	*Assumptions of the Holistic Model*
Treatment of symptoms	Search for patterns, causes
Specialized	Integrated, concerned with the whole patient
Emphasis on efficiency	Emphasis on human values
Professional should be emotionally neutral	Professional's caring is a component of healing
Pain and disease are wholly negative	Pain and disease may be valuable signals of internal conflicts
Primary intervention with drugs, surgery	Minimal intervention with appropriate technology, complemented with full armamentarium of noninvasive techniques (psychotechnologies, diet, exercise)
Body seen as machine in good or bad repair	Body seen as dynamic system, a complex energy field within fields (family, workplace, environment, culture, life history)
Disease or disability seen as entity	Disease or disability seen as process
Emphasis on eliminating symptoms, disease	Emphasis on achieving maximum bodymind health
Patient is dependent	Patient is (or should be) autonomous
Professional is authority	Professional is therapeutic partner
Body and mind are separate: psychosomatic illnesses seen as mental; may refer to psychiatrist	Bodymind perspective: psychosomatic illness is the province of all health-care professionals
Mind is secondary factor in organic illness	Mind is primary or co-equal factor in all illness
Placebo effect is evidence of power of suggestion	Placebo effect is evidence of mind's role in disease and healing
Primary reliance on quantitative information (charts, tests, dates)	Primary reliance on qualitative information, including patient reports and professional's intuition; quantitative data an adjunct
"Prevention" seen as largely environmental: vitamins, rest, exercise, immunization, not smoking	"Prevention" synonymous with wholeness: in work, relationships, goals, body-mind-spirit

SOURCE: *The Aquarian Conspiracy: Personal and Social Transformations in the 1980's*, © 1980 by Marilyn Ferguson, published by J. P. Tarcher, Inc., Houghton Mifflin (9110 Sunset Boulevard, Los Angeles, Calif. 90069), pp. 246–248. Used by permission.

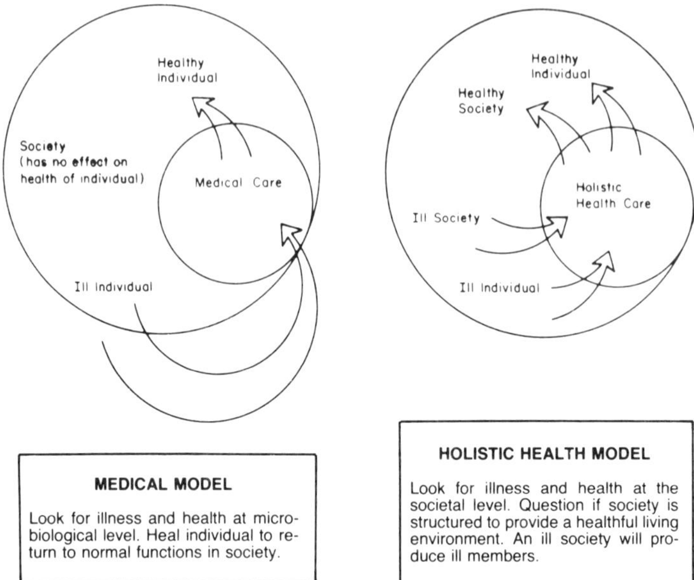

Figure 2-1. Relationship between the individual and society in two medical models. [SOURCE: David Hayes-Bautista and Dominic S. Harveston, "Holistic Health Care," *Social Policy* (March/April, 1977), pp. 7–13. © 1977 by Social Policy Corporation, 33 West 42nd Street, New York, N.Y. 10036. Used by permission.]

> doctor, according to this view, is essentially a mechanic who patches up the body after it has been damaged by illness or injury.[14]

Frank believes that while modern medicine has produced dazzling triumphs, it fails to consider the individual as a psychobiological unit, "a total being whose thoughts, perceptions, and feelings are intimately connected with his biochemistry and physiology." This concept of human being as a psychobiological unit is at the heart of holistic theory: a healthy person is one whose total system—both mind and body—is in a state of dynamic equilibrium in which healing or restorative functions are stronger than pathogenic or destructive ones. Illness results when pathogenic forces prevail. Healing occurs when a healthy equilibrium is restored either spontaneously or with the aid of a medical or nonmedical healer.[15] Holistic health approaches focusing

[14]Jerome D. Frank, "The Medical Power of Faith," *Human Nature* (August, 1978), pp. 40ff.

[15]*Ibid.*

on the individual include spiritual, psychological, and physical health modalities or therapies; among these are such techniques as T'ai Chi, yoga, EST, dance therapy, bioenergetics, Rolfing, acupuncture, and other less well-known techniques (see Appendices B & C, pages 29–37).

The holistic health movement has a significant and growing following. Milton Friedman, a journalist and congressional staffperson, has estimated that 2 million people are involved in personal, inner-growth approaches to health. Other commentators estimate that 5 million Americans now ascribe to the lifestyle termed "voluntary simplicity," which is associated with both personal and environmental approaches to health.[16] The large number of joggers and other exercise enthusiasts appears to corroborate this trend.

James Turner, author of *The Chemical Feast*,[17] stated (see Chapter 1) that the pharmaceutical industry is in its death throes because many people are "voting with their feet" for a growing range of alternative therapies (see Appendices B & C). The bases of many of the alternative therapies proposed by the holistic health movement differ from those of allopathic medicine. Before considering the implications of increased interest in holistic therapies on federal policy toward pharmaceutical R & D, these assumptions should be examined.

COMPARING TREATMENT MODALITIES

The existence of a wide range of alternative therapies raises questions about their comparative contributions to health. The question of comparative efficacy cannot yet be answered because of inadequate systematic research on the success of individual therapies. Like most others, therapists in the new modalities shun systematic research on treatment outcomes. They have been able to do so because they are not subject to FDA safety and efficacy standards and because there has been little market pressure for them to submit to systematic evaluation.

One issue that has been raised is a sensitive one for many holistic practitioners: who is to decide which therapies are "good"? Many participants in alternative therapies view pressure for objective evalu-

[16]Duane Elgin and Arnold Mitchell, "Voluntary Simplicity," *Co-evolution Quarterly* (Summer, 1977), pp. 4–19.

[17]James Turner, *The Chemical Feast: Nader Report on the Food and Drug Administration*, (New York: Penguin, 1977).

ation as an attempt to force new therapies into a preconceived mold. Practitioners of alternative therapies will undoubtedly develop their own standards of therapeutic efficacy. However, these standards will probably vary from school to school: each has different notions about the nature of illness and is likely to accept different criteria as proof of efficacy.

In the United States, homeopathy is an alternative, if not a "new," health technology, practiced by some 1,500 medical doctors. It is far more widespread in India and much of Europe. Its assumptions about the nature of disease differ radically from those of allopathic medicine. Homeopathic practitioners believe that illness represents a disturbance in a vital life force. Symptoms of illness are looked upon as the body's natural process of shrugging off the disturbance. Because therapies are designed to further this process by "drawing out" the symptoms, a homeopathy patient might experience a temporary worsening of symptoms during the course of therapy.

According to homeopathic theory, the more a substance is diluted, the more powerful its effects will be. Theoretically, then, a medication can be diluted to a point where no drug is present and still be therapeutically effective. This notion stands in direct contradiction to modern principles of pharmacology.[18]

Acupuncture is another example of an alternative health modality. Although it is a "new" health technology in the United States, acupuncture has a tradition far older than allopathic medicine. Acupuncture points are located on meridians along with "Ch'i energy" flows. The existence of Ch'i energy is an underlying assumption of the major health modality of the world's largest nation, the People's Republic of China, yet it is not recognized by American science or medicine. Research has shown that acupuncture points have elevated levels of radioactivity and that skin surrounding these points has a measurable level of extra electrical conductivity.[19] Nevertheless, the manner in which acupuncture works has not yet been scientifically substantiated.

The use of behavioral techniques for treating hypertension is another example of an alternative health technology. According to small-scale clinical studies, biofeedback, Zen meditation, and related

[18]Harris Livermore Coulter, *Divided Legacy: A History of the Schism in Medical Thought*, Vol. 3, *Science and Ethics in American Medicine, 1800–1914* (Washington, D.C.: Wehawken Book Company, 1973), pp. 57, 491–492.

[19]Robert M. Duggan, "An Overview of Completed Research on Acupuncture," *Journal of Traditional Acupuncture*, Vol. 2 (Summer, 1978), pp. 43–50.

techniques have some efficacy in lowering blood pressure. However, more extensive clinical testing is needed before useful conclusions about efficacy can be drawn.[20]

Many holistic health modalities serve as avenues to personal inner growth rather than as remedies for specific ailments. However, some of these modalities may indeed have therapeutic value. Herbert Benson describes a "relaxation response" that results from spiritual/religious exercises and transcendental and other forms of meditation. Theoretically, this relaxation response could benefit an insomniac by eliminating underlying stress rather than by dealing directly with symptoms of sleeplessness.[21]

THE ROLE OF THE FEDERAL GOVERNMENT IN PHARMACEUTICAL R & D

The advent of alternative approaches to health care raises questions about the role of the federal government as a promoter and regulator of new therapies, particularly drugs. Legislators may be called upon to reassess the therapeutic and social costs and benefits of the allopathic approach to health care.

To promote the most productive pharmaceutical research, federal regulatory policy might be redesigned to identify and encourage R & D in areas where drug therapy clearly continues to be preferred. It may become necessary to formulate new operational definitions of safety and efficacy and to determine whether these definitions can be applied to alternative health care systems. If medical insurance plans pay for health care from non-M.D. providers, legislators may have to consider the effect of such coverage on market demand for pharmaceuticals and the consequent targeting of industry R & D effort.

Many of those involved in the holistic health movement do not believe that the government should play a significant role in the promotion of new therapies. Rather, they believe that "personal health consciousness" will advance the holistic health movement. According to Milton Friedman:

> healing . . . that flows from a different level of consciousness cannot be legislated into existence by a government that clings to conventional fixations. In the immediate future, those seeking healing will find it in themselves and not in some massive new federal program that imposes

[20] Alvin P. Shapiro *et al.*, "Behavioral Methods in Treatment of Hypertension: Review of Their Clinical Status," *Annals of Internal Medicine* (forthcoming).

[21] Herbert Benson, *The Relaxation Response* (New York: William Morrow, 1975).

> universal salvation from Washington. . . . The answer to the holistic question cannot come from presidential commissions or acts of Congress. . . . It is within the willingness of the individual to become holistically responsible.[22]

Friedman does not call for a cessation of government activity in the health area nor does he call for a halt to the development of new pharmaceutical therapies. He maintains, however, the wellness can be facilitated but not developed by the government and that most government policy is based on the doctor-as-intervenor assumption of allopathic medicine.

Current federal drug regulatory policy is built either explicitly or implicitly on several assumptions. Policymakers recognize that the allopathic school of medicine is the major approach to treatment in our society. The public requires allopathic drugs that are highly effective for specific illness when prescribed appropriately by physicians. The individual physician needs assurance from an objective third party (such as the FDA) that the drugs he or she prescribes are safe, effective, and manufactured under strict quality control standards. Because third parties regulate drug utilization through "access to market" control, the need for doctors to maintain records on the efficacy of the drugs they prescribe and the need for systematic rational data gathering on drug safety and efficacy are neglected.

Health policymakers further assume that scientifically sound measures of safety and efficacy can be determined by clinical research on a relatively small number of humans before a drug is marketed. Moreover, there is no requirement that regulatory agencies compare the efficacy of similar types of drugs or of various treatment modalities.

The increased use of alternative therapies indicates that these assumptions are being questioned by a growing number of health care providers and consumers. Future policy choices may go beyond the narrowly defined regulatory function presently assumed by the government in regard to pharmaceuticals. Legislators may be called upon to increase the awareness among providers and consumers of alternative health care modalities and to promote greater equality of access to the market for competing therapies. Appendix A (below) outlines some of the proposed policy options for regulating drugs in light of the rise of alternative therapies.

[22] Milton Friedman, "Holistic Health: Is Washington Listening?" *New Realities*, Vol. 11, No. 1, p. 20.

APPENDIX A

Policy Options for Regulating Safety and Efficacy of New Drugs in Light of the Growing Popularity of Alternative Therapies

---

I. Premarketing policy options for assuring safety and efficacy
   A. Make market access easier
      1. Decrease amount of animal testing necessary
      2. Decrease amount of human testing necessary
      3. Ease premarket definitions of safety and efficacy allowing greater postmarket surveillance
      4. Ease efficacy requirements and allow the market to determine these
      5. Allow greater use of foreign data on safety and efficacy
      6. Modify current requirements for adequate and well-controlled studies to permit consideration of additional evidence in the form of:
         a. Well-documented controlled studies reported in reputable medical journals
         b. Opinions of expert panels (NAS/NRC review—OTC review
   B. Make market access more difficult
      1. Develop standards of comparative safety and efficacy for drugs with the same purpose
      2. Develop standards of comparative safety and efficacy for therapies used for the same purpose

II. Postmarketing policy options for monitoring safety and efficacy
   A. Keep record of anticipated new uses
   B. Establish patterns of use
   C. Identify side effects

III. Options for promoting effective utilization of drugs
   A. Increase information availability
      1. Develop national information system for collecting data on therapeutic effects of drugs in use
      2. Develop national information system for collecting data on therapeutic effects of all health modalities in use

3. Develop multiple sources, e.g., AMA, Consumers Union, Medical Letter, or Commonweal to use national data to evaluate and recommend therapies of choice for specified conditions

B. Increase information dissemination
   1. Equalize access to communications channels
      a. Require various sides to be presented
         (1) Provide patient package insert
         (2) Include data on comparative efficacy in presentations by "detail persons"
      b. Facilitate the presentation of alternative positions
         (1) Fund counterdetail persons
         (2) Fund counteradvertising
   2. Identify other major information sources physicians use to learn about drugs and ensure equal access

C. Alter physician learning incentives
   1. Require continuing education that includes comparative efficacy of therapies in use
   2. Require physician recordkeeping on drug prescribing, costs, and effects
   3. Establish more local utilization review committees of physicians
      a. To review federal drug reimbursement programs
      b. Part of the responsibility of all those who prescribe drugs

D. Increase the number of persons able to prescribe drugs
   1. Establish a schedule of drugs based on level of technical training necessary for prescribing
   2. License pharmacists, nurse-practitioners, and others to prescribe drugs
   3. Eliminate prescription requirements altogether

APPENDIX B

Health Modality Matrix

Richard Miles, Dean of the Graduate Program in Holistic Health Education at John F. Kennedy University in Olinda, California, has prepared the following matrix of health modalities. It is particularly relevant for considering the implications of the holistic health movement for pharmaceutical R & D for two reasons: (1) its placement of orthodox drug treatment within physical disciplines that take a biochemical approach to health and (2) the standards by which health modalities are differentiated and evaluated.

Miles asserts that true health emerges as a by-product of the individual's efforts to integrate three aspects of change through a personally designed blend of disciplines that offer life purpose, expression, and movement. The three aspects are (1) recognizing unproductive patterns of action, (2) achieving short- and long-term physical homeostasis (relaxing, rebalancing, and detoxifying the body), and (3) replacing unwanted behavior with purposeful patterns through new goals, strategies, and actions.

In presenting this matrix, Miles adds comments that are particularly relevant to our discussion:

1. Quality assurance in any modality can be accomplished only through consumer awareness, wise buying, and effective feedback mechanisms reporting outcome.
2. The success of any consumer integration of a life health plan using several disciplines based on awareness of goals is more a function of that awareness than of the efficacy of any discipline.
3. Professional peer review within any discipline accomplishes only the control of entry and practice and usually has no outcome measurement component.
4. The baseline essential change in new health perspectives is the giving up of the assumption by the technological world of a hostile environment and adopting a belief system more in resonance with an essentially friendly universe; i.e., the unproductive patterns, when recognized, are frequently based on unnecessary self-protection.

Appendix B. Health Modality Matrix

	Diagnosis: Recognition & Evaluation Patterns of Behavior	*Techniques for Achieving Homeostasis: Relaxation, Rebalancing, & Detoxification*	*Providing Personal Goals: Purpose, Strategy, and/or Action*
I. Spiritual disciplines—deal with the person's image of self and relation to the universe			
1. Dream work	Dream journal	Realization of meaning and conflict	Dream guidance
2. Inner guide imagery	Question formulation	Meditation, visualization	Inner guidance
3. Jungian symbolism	Review of personal symbolism	Realization of meaning and acceptance of conflict	Insight into inner wisdom
4. Logotherapy	Review of search for meaning	Realization of meaning and acceptance of conflict	Insight into inner wisdom
5. Psychosynthesis	Review of subpersonalities, higher self	Meditation, visualization	Integration of will and purpose
6. Tai Chi Chuan	Assessment of relationship to balance, energies	Meditation, movement awareness, focus	Integration of life energies
7. Yoga	Recognition of mind/body/attitude patterns	Focus, postures, structural awareness	Integration of life energies

II. Psychological disciplines—deal with life strategies at the level of mind (but usually not spirit)			
A. Mind systems—coping strategies only			
1. Behavior modification	Behavior analysis		New behavior
2. Mind trainings a. Actualizations b. est c. Mind dynamics d. Silva mind control	Confrontation of behavior patterns	(This aspect not seriously dealt with by any of the mind/strategy disciplines)	New strategies of interaction (politics of the facade)
3. Psychoanalysis	Identification of labelled patterns		New behavior
B. Psycho-physical disciplines—deal with mind/body coordination and the relationship of strategy to physical effects			
1. Alexander	Review of eye-body action patterns	Movement and exercise/breathing	New flexibility
2. Arica Psycho-calisthenics	Awareness of range of motion	Movement and exercise/breathing	New flexibility
3. Biofeedback	Awareness of action patterns	Progressive relaxation techniques	New patterns
4. Biorhythms	Chart development	Acceptance of natural patterns	Calendar phase planning of action
5. Dance therapy	None	Movement/breathing	New flexibility
6. Guided imagery	Identification of issue to be changed	Progressive relaxation	Change in physical pattern
7. Feldenkrais	None	Movement/breathing	New range of motion

Appendix B. (Continued)

	Diagnosis: Recognition & Evaluation Patterns of Behavior	Techniques for Achieving Homeostasis: Relaxation, Rebalancing, & Detoxification	Providing Personal Goals: Purpose, Strategy, and/or Action
C. Emotional/physical disciplines—seek to treat pain and augment body resistance by counteracting the body's "blocks," or physiological changes that result from negative emotional events			
1. Bioenergetics	Identification of emotional body patterns	Movement/breathing	Release of body energy
2. Gestalt (could be under psychophysical)	Identification of parts and wholes, polarities	Resolution of conflict	Experiencing here and now
3. Primal therapy	Identification of early life trauma	Clearing through re-experience	Release of energy
4. Reichian	Identification of emotional blocks	Clearing through intense experience	Release of energy
5. Sensitivity training	Identification of fears and phobias	Clearing through intense experience	Freedom from phobias
6. Sexuality training	Identification of fears and blocks	Clearing through awareness and experience	Greater sexual expression
III. Physical disciplines—change through the body directly			
A. Structural/muscular			
1. Bates eye (developmental vision therapy)	Check vision	Exercises	Improved vision
2. Chiropractic	Check spinal alignment	Alignment	Improved neural function

3. Kinesiology (related to metabolic and etheric)	Check muscular strength	Rebalance energy	Improved function
4. Osteopathy	Check structural alignment	Adjust structure	Improved function
5. Structural integration a. Postural b. Rolfing c. Trager	Check structural alignment, muscular imbalance	Adjust structure	Improved function, released tension
	(These practices can be expanded by the practitioner to include psycho-physical and emotional-physical outcomes of new strategies and energy release)		
6. Temporomandibular joint technique	Check jaw alignment	Adjust structure	Released tension, improved function
7. Yoga (when practiced only as physical exercise)	Awareness of structural/muscular facility	Exercises, postures	Released tension, improved function
B. Biochemical			
1. Homeopathy	Case analysis	Remedy matching symptoms	Facilitate self-healing
2. Allopathy	Case analysis	Remedy opposing symptoms (does not relax, rebalance, or detoxify)	Eliminate disease symptoms
C. Metabolic			
Orthomolecular, megavitamin, and nutrition therapies	Hair analysis, nutrition analysis, blood tests	Chelation, colonic therapies, megavitamins, minerals, enzymes	Rebalance metabolism

Appendix B. (Continued)

	Diagnosis: Recognition & Evaluation Patterns of Behavior	*Techniques for Achieving Homeostasis: Relaxation, Rebalancing, & Detoxification*	*Providing Personal Goals: Purpose, Strategy, and/or Action*
D. Etheric (or body energy)			
1. Acupuncture	Pulse diagnosis	Rebalance energy	Homeostasis of energy
2. Ryoduraku acup	Chart of meridians	Rebalance energy	Homeostasis of energy
3. Acupressure Systems	Energy imbalance	Rebalance energy	Homeostasis of energy
a. Polarity therapy			
b. Kinesiology			
c. Jin Shin Jyutsu			
d. Shiatsu			
e. Reflexology			
4. Kirlian photo	Energy flow analysis	None	None
5. Psychic	Aura/energy visualization	Varies with practitioner	Symptom relief, energy rebalance
IV. Analagous or diagnostic systems			
1. Iridology	Analysis of iris patterns	None	None
2. Palmistry	Analysis of hand patterns	None	None
3. Personology	Analysis of body ratios, characteristics, shapes	None	Awareness of structural tendencies for life actions
4. Graphology	Analysis of handwriting	None	Awareness of personality characteristics

SOURCE: Richard B. Miles, "Health Modality Matrix," Holistic Health Program, John F. Kennedy University, San Francisco, Calif. (Presented to Commonweal/OTA Conference on New Technologies and Health, Bolinas, Calif., November 19–20, 1978). Used with permission.

APPENDIX C

New Health Care Technologies[23]

I. Environment and health
  A. Environmentally induced disease
  B. Environmental design and health promotion
    1. Workplace environment
    2. Safety or toxicity of building material
    3. Health considerations in the design of buildings and communities
    4. Health and light
    5. Noise as an environmental stressor
    6. The use of color to promote health
    7. Air ions and health

II. Physiology and health
  A. Nutritional/metabolic techniques
    1. Clinical ecology
    2. The Feingold diet
    3. Orthomolecular medicine
    4. The Airola diet
    5. The Pritikin program
    6. Plant and herbal medicine
  B. Fitness and movement
    1. Sports medicine
    2. Fitness programs
    3. Sensory awareness
    4. Bio-energetics
    5. Dance
    6. Martial arts
  C. Physical manipulation
    1. Chiropractic
    2. Applied kinesiology
    3. Temporomandibular joint technique (TMJ)
    4. Massage
    5. Shiatsu
    6. Polarity therapy
    7. Alexander technique

[23]Rick J. Carlson and the Commonweal Research Institute Staff, "Preliminary Report to the Office of Technology Assessment on New Health Care Technologies" (Bolinas, Calif.: Commonweal Research Institute, 1978), pp. 27–28.

        8. Rolfing
        9. Feldenkrais
        10. Lomi
    D. Acupuncture and acupuncture-related techniques
    E. Electromagnetic therapies
    F. Developmental vision therapy (Bates method)
III. Technique for health appraisal and assessment
    A. Health decision-making tools
    B. Health hazard appraisal
    C. Health risk appraisal
IV. Mind/body interaction
    A. Biofeedback
    B. Relaxation techniques
        1. Autogenic training
    C. Imagery and suggestion
        1. Hypnosis
        2. Therapeutic use of placebo
        3. Visualization as a therapeutic tool
        4. Suggestion and disease
    D. Meditation/yoga
    E. Laying on of hands
        1. Therapeutic touch
        2. All nonmanipulative techniques working with the body
V. Diagnostic techniques
    A. Iridiology
    B. Reflexology
    C. Pulse diagnosis
    D. Hair analysis for minerals and toxic metals
VI. Ethnomedicine
VII. Integrated systems of new technologies for health promotion
    A. Self-help/self-care
        1. Self-directed and administered
        2. Self-initiated
    B. Behavior modification techniques
        1. Smoking
        2. Weight loss
        3. Fitness
        4. Dietary alteration
    C. Biological rhythms
    D. Life cycle management
        1. Birthing

   2. Death and dying
   3. Aging
   4. Human sexuality
   5. Life stages
  E. Family and group work
  F. Psycho-cybernetics
   1. est
   2. ARICA, etc.
  G. Hospices and other programs dealing with death and dying
  H. Birthing centers
VIII. Other systems of medicine

HIGHLIGHTS OF THE DISCUSSION

An important concern in the field of health care is the extent to which current medicine is holistic, allopathic, scientific, or ascientific. The problem of determining which modality best characterizes modern medicine is complicated by the difficulty of talking across paradigms or schools of thought. A paradigm or model either explicitly or implicitly structures reality for its user: in research, including medical research, it identifies relevant questions as well as ways to judge the answers to those questions. Those within a particular paradigm may not even recognize that they are operating within it. To the extent that there is a dominant paradigm in current medical practice, it is placed historically in the reductionist, allopathic approach.

Murray Weiner, research vice president at the Merrell Research Center, challenged the use of the term *allopathic medicine.* According to Weiner, the distinction between homeopathy and allopathy meant something 150 years ago. Modern medicine, he claimed, has little to do with either philosophy. Medicine as it is practiced today is grounded in science. Whether the philosophy is homeopathy, surgery, manipulative physiotherapy, ying/yang balance, or meditation, a technique becomes of interest to the practicing physician when sound scientific evidence is developed to demonstrate its practical worth. It is, therefore, an error to enumerate a long list of spiritual, psychological, and physical "treatment modalities" and imply that so-called allopathic medicine is just one more "treatment modality" that happens to have a high acceptance right now but may deserve to be downgraded in favor of other disciplines.

Medical practice is continuously changing. Mistakes are made, and there is a continuing need for criticism and correction. It would be a tragic mistake for society if the subtle undercurrent of antiscience now sweeping our country were to reach into the practice of medicine and fragment health care into competing "treatment modalities" based on competing philosophies rather than on knowledge and the general laws of nature, Weiner said. Concepts currently labeled holistic have been fundamental medical teaching long before the word became popular. What is most troublesome about the current system is the physician's inability to use fully his or her holistic judgments to each patient's advantage because of the yes/no demand for yes/no proof of safety and efficacy. But to deny a prime place to scientific concepts and the enormously successful pharmaceutical advances of recent decades is to undermine rather than promote what is real and practical in the holistic movement.

Furthermore, he added, the physician has an obligation to treat sickness regardless of what produces it—whether it is the organism or society or both. While research seeks to prevent or cure illnesses, there will always be disease that remains, and it falls to the doctor to treat those who do become sick. Wipe out one of the 10 leading causes of death, and number 11 would move up. Young people who would have died of diphtheria or polio if there were no vaccines are now living to suffer coronary or lung disease for which we continuously seek a more effective spectrum of new medications. If we conquered lung cancer or cardiovascular disease, people would die of something else, and there will remain an unending need for pharmaceutical R & D to help control that something else. It is in the public interest to keep pharmaceutical R & D healthy. Even if federal support extends to nontraditional approaches in medicine, such approaches should not distract from the development of pharmaceutical therapies. In fact, the government should lessen disincentives created by unnecessary, ineffective, and increasingly detailed regulations, he concluded.

Rick Carlson, author of *The End of Medicine*, argued that holism is not an either/or proposition and is compatible with medicine. He agreed with Weiner that more research about holistic health techniques is needed but felt it important to note that holism is not the summation of various new health techniques. Holism is a belief system. Its power lies in the way we think about ourselves as human beings and the institutions we create as an outgrowth of this. And although much scientific research is needed in the area of holistic health practices, it is worth noting that modern medicine is ascientific in many aspects because it is more involved with process than with outcome.

Carlson claimed that growth in the medical care system has been determined more by political and economic factors than by its relationship to therapeutic outcomes and predicted increased political pressure from holistic practitioners who want to be incorporated into mainstream medicine and a reallocation of government resources as recognition of the many determinants of health grows. He proposed seven assumptions about health and the health care system that form the basis of his ideas about the use of alternative therapies.

1. The medical system will change only when society as a whole changes. Therefore, in discussing the future of the medical care system, we must talk about the future and values of society as a whole.

2. Holism is not various techniques or modalities or the sum of such techniques. The concept of holism is a very profound one as an antidote to excessively reductionist thinking about who we are as human animals and about how the institutions we have today ought to change as we move into the future.

3. Holistic thinking is being applied vigorously to the medical care system because our approach to health through medicine is the most reductionist of the scientific disciplines and must be at dissonance with who we are as human beings and who we think we ought to be. There is a movement toward "naturalness" in products and services that will be very important for medicine and pharmaceuticals.

4. Many of the "new techniques" will lose appeal over time. They are first-generational attempts at something profound. Over the next 10 years, basic biomedical research should include extensive research into the capacity of the human organism for self-regulation. These new technologies are but precursors of self-regulatory technologies that will emerge.

5. The entire attempt to deal with health problems by suppressing symptoms is fundamentally wrong. Ultimately, the most profound therapeutic approach may be to allow individuals to express the symptomology of the experience that we call disease. In order for an individual to learn from the experience, the disease process must go through several stages of expression. Premature suppression of symptoms defers the problem.

6. There is an impulse, perhaps even an instinct, in the human being to ingest chemicals such as drugs, alcohol, and caffeine to alter the sense of consciousness.

7. The medical system and pharmaceutical enterprises exist primarily for political, economic, and social reasons not therapeutic ones. The health care industry, like the petrochemical industry and others, exists because that is the way we do things. The health care system has an important employment function that is not necessarily related to its therapeutic function.

Although Carlson agreed that to attack allopathic medicine per se is to miss the point, he noted that premature suppression of symptomology is at the base of allopathy's theory of healing. He emphasized that it is the medical system, its institutional forms, and its theory of healing that must be examined.

Shelia Touquan of the pharmaceutical program of the Blue Cross and Blue Shield Associations felt that holism is not opposed to the allopathic model. Rather, subspecialization has taken much of the "care out of the cure," and holism is attempting to put the care back in.

Holism is traditional medicine practiced in a modern environment, she explained. The holistic model will eventually be institutionalized, and people will go to these centers for both their physical and emotional health needs—much like an HMO (Health Maintenance Organization). Patients will receive health care not only from physicians but from counselors and clergy as well, she claimed. Finally, holism leads to a recognition that the individual must play a more active role in his/her own health. Insurance companies are now encouraging this through mechanisms such as reduced premiums for nonsmokers and the physically fit.

Carlson countered her argument by noting that, with the exception of certain proven techniques such as biofeedback, holistic modalities are not amenable to reimbursement. Thus, access to most of these modalities will be limited to those with the time and money to take advantage of them. Moreover, federal regulation of the new approaches could strangle holism.

3
The Effect of Regulation on Incentives for Pharmaceutical R & D

The incentives for pharmaceutical companies to engage in the discovery, development, and introduction of new drugs to market have received much attention because of a decline in research productivity as measured by the output of new chemical entities. The increasing cost and time involved in taking a drug to the marketplace (now estimated at $54 million and up to 10 years) also call attention to incentives. Much analysis during the last 10 years has attributed these decreasing incentives to the burden placed on pharmaceutical companies by FDA regulation, particularly as mandated in the 1962 amendments to the 1938 federal Food, Drug, and Cosmetic Act. In fact, the most recent analysis of Henry Grabowski of Duke University suggests that regulation was responsible for about one-third of the increase in cost between 1960 and 1975. Attention has also been focused on other factors that may have increased the cost of drug innovation, including increasing health care costs, new analytic techniques for measuring the safety and efficacy of drugs, increasing concern for safety on the part of drug companies, and depletion of research opportunities.

More recent analyses by investment specialists have identified favorable changes in the FDA's approach since 1976 as well as significant market success of certain new drugs. While it is suggested that annual global sales for a new product have to reach $10 to $12 million to make the development of the product economically feasible, a few new drugs have significantly exceeded these annual sales figures. These factors raise important questions about the incentives for pharmaceutical companies, the market, and the impact of government regulation.

INCENTIVES FOR PHARMACEUTICAL FIRMS

Pharmaceutical firms are the only organizations that develop new drugs expressly for marketing and are one of the major sources of research to discover new drugs. In examining regulation and its influence on incentives, it is useful to distinguish between research-intensive firms and nonresearch-intensive firms. A recent study identified 25 research-intensive firms and 24 nonresearch-intensive firms.[1]

The 25 research-intensive firms had an average of nearly $400 million in global sales and committed an average of $37.5 million to their global R & D activities. The 24 nonresearch-intensive firms had global sales averaging $52 million and spent only $2.9 million on R & D. The research-intensive firms spent the equivalent of 9.4% of their sales on R & D.

Pharmaceutical firms are science and technology dependent organizations operating in various markets and submarkets. As such they have scientific as well as intra-organizational incentives for advancing the state of what is known.[2] However, firms are often looked upon as "rational actors" presumed to follow economic incentives. Thus, economic incentives have received the most attention.

The major reason for research-intensive pharmaceutical firms to reinvest 9% or 10% of their sales in research is to maintain or enhance their ability to market new drugs. New drugs can be placed in three categories: (1) "orphan" or "service" drugs that are developed for other than immediate economic reasons, (2) drugs that will yield sales sufficient to justify the research and development investment (current industry discussion suggests this requires $10 to $12 million in annual global sales, usually allowing 3 to 5 years after introduction to build a market), and (3) bonanza or "jackpot" drugs whose global sales exceed $100 million annually.

When a typical pharmaceutical company explores its opportunities, first a research-planner or research vice president receives a market analysis that provides estimates of the third- or fifth-year potential sales of a drug with certain characteristics. The number of physician visits and type of prescriptions that may be written for a given condi-

[1]Fay Dworkin, "Impact of Disclosure of Safety and Efficacy Data on Expenditures for Pharmaceutical Research and Development" (Washington, D.C.: Food and Drug Administration, April, 1978).

[2]Graham T. Allison, *The Essence of Decision* (Boston: Little Brown, 1971); Richard E. Faust, "Project Selection in the Pharmaceutical Industry," *Research Management*, Vol. 14, No. 5 (September, 1971), pp. 46–55.

tion is forecast as well as the potential market for specific new chemical entities or modifications of existing drugs. Financial incentives are determined for pursuing new drugs for diseases or conditions of high incidence as well as for drugs that improve existing products by offering greater patient convenience, by reducing or eliminating the level of toxic reactions of currently available drugs, by providing a less frequent or lower cost regimen, by providing a more effective mode of action, or by serving a broader range of people with the particular disease.

When forecast of sales is complete, decisionmakers match the company's resources (scientific personnel, plant and equipment, and experience) to those needed to discover or develop the potential drug. If the research involves a new molecular entity, the research-planner must estimate the likelihood of discovery of a molecular entity with the desired therapeutic effect and minimal or acceptable side effects. A significant part of the decision to pursue a project involves judgments about the costs of discovering and taking the drug to the marketplace.

It is important to note that several areas of government policy other than regulation also affect a company's incentives for R & D. Patents, for example, allow a company exclusive rights to the commercial use of a product it discovers for a period of 17 years. A standard assumption is that patents are necessary. Since the information required to discover a new drug is costly to produce but relatively inexpensive to copy, patents are needed to induce innovation.[3] Some industry spokespeople have argued for an increase in the life of a patent because of the time lost for development, testing, and FDA approval. Other economists, however, have suggested that the industry would innovate even without patents, since competition in the drug industry results from innovation rather than from price competition.[4] Still other economists have argued that patents are necessary, although patent life should be reduced.[5]

[3]Howard I. Forman, "Patents, Compulsory Licensing, Prices and Innovation," *The Proceedings of the First Seminar on Economics of Pharmaceutical Innovation*, ed. Joseph D. Cooper (Washington, D.C.: The American University, 1970), pp. 177–195; E. Jucker, *Patents Why?* (Basel, Switzerland: Buchdruckerei Gasser & Cie, 1972).

[4]William S. Comanor, "Research and Competitive Product Differentiation in the Pharmaceutical Industry in the United States," *Economica* Vol. 31 (November, 1964), pp. 372–384.

[5]Leonard G. Schifrin, "The Ethical Drug Industry: The Case of Compulsory Patent Licensing," *Antitrust Bulletin*, Vol. 12 (Fall, 1967), pp. 893–915.

COSTS AND BENEFITS OF DISCOVERING AND DEVELOPING A NEW DRUG

In 1970 Harold Clymer estimated that it took 5 to 7 years and cost $3 to $5 million to develop a single marketed product. He also noted that, in terms of company economics, the successful drug must carry the costs of failures, that is, the 80% of compounds for which testing was initiated but abandoned (see Figure 3-1).

From 1962 to 1972, development costs per new chemical entity (NCE) rose from $1.2 to $11.5 million. According to the University of Rochester, the most recent estimate of development costs, including the opportunity cost of capital, reaches $7.7 million for the successful NCE itself and another $16.3 million for the failures, bringing the total to $24 million. (See the work of pharmacologist Leon Goldberg,[6] Chapter 1, and Figure 1-1 for additional information on the process of drug development.)

A recent extensive study by Ronald Hansen on the cost of the R & D process surveyed 65 drugs that reflected about 10% of all drugs tested by 25 firms over a 10-year period. It was found that 1 in 8 drugs that began the testing process ultimately made it to the market.[7] Other estimates have varied from 1 to 6[8] to 1 in 22.[9] Hansen arrived at the figure of $54 million of total investment required to discover and develop the average new drug in 1976.

This $54 million included $30 million for research and $24 million for development. The $24 million included $5.7 million to test the average successful NCE, $11.3 million for developmental work on the seven compounds that began testing but were dropped along the way, and $7.3 million for the opportunity costs figured at 8% of development expenditures. While the success ratio for the development stage in Hansen's sample was 1 compound in 8, for the discovery stage it may have been 1 in 1,000 or more. Thus, it is not possible to isolate the discovery costs of the successful NCEs using the

[6]Leon I. Goldberg, "Creativity in Drug Development: An Academic Challenge," *Perspectives in Biology and Medicine* (Winter, 1978), pp. 188–195.

[7]Ronald W. Hansen, "The Pharmaceutical Development Process: Estimates of Current Costs and Times and the Effects of Regulatory Changes, Paper GPB 77-10" (University of Rochester Center for Research in Government Policy and Business, revised July, 1978).

[8]Harold A. Clymer, "The Economics of Drug Innovation," *The Development and Control of New Products*, eds. M. Pernarowski and M. Darrach (Vancouver: University of British Columbia).

[9]William W. Wardell and Louis Lasagna, *Regulation and Drug Development* (Washington, D.C.: American Enterprise Institute, 1975).

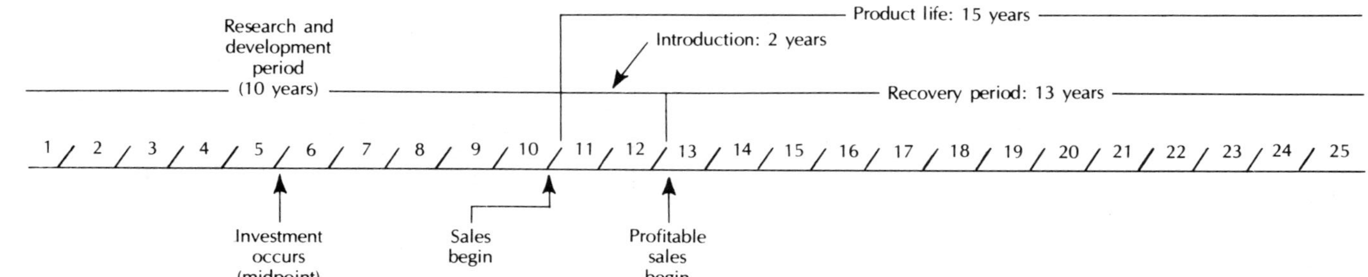

Figure 3-1. Time periods from research to marketing of a new drug product. [SOURCE: Harold A. Clymer, "The Economics of Drug Innovation," *The Development and Control of New Products,* eds. M. Pernarowski and M. Darrach (Vancouver: University of British Columbia), p. 123. Used by permission.]

data from Hansen's studies. Hansen estimated an average discovery cost by dividing the total research expenditures by the number of successful NCEs. Using this approach he found that the discovery expenditures were approximately $16 million per successful NCE. The remaining $14 million of the $30 million discovery figure is the 8% return on investment in research activities made 6 to 10 years before the successful NCE is marketed.

Figure 3-2 breaks down the $5.7 million in development costs for the average successful NCE using the timeline from Figure 3-1. Amounts in parentheses represent capitalization of the expenses of that phase of development for a total of $7.7 million to develop a successful NCE including the cost of the initial investment.

As noted, some research planners feel that sales forecasts of $10 to $12 million in annual global sales are necessary to make a drug worth developing. In many cases, it appears that drug firms set their sights even higher. According to one analyst, 12 of the drugs marketed since 1963 have had estimated annual wordwide sales of $150 million or more. The leaders of this group are Valium and the recently marketed ulcer drug, Tagamet (see Table 3-1). The practice of looking for a large-volume drug has prompted a comparison of the drug industry to the oil industry, which sinks wells in search of a potentially rich return.[10] This explains why some firms continue to invest in research despite the small number of profitable new drugs that are actually discovered.[11]

Investment analyst David Saks claims, "Because of the great successes of new drugs such as Motrin, Tagamet, and Clinoril, allocations for research funding are being substantially increased relative to the past" (see Table 3-2).[12] It should be noted, however, that a major research cost is salaries and wages. Since this single factor has been increasing at about 8% per year, the real growth in research activity is substantially less than indicated in Table 3-2. In addition, rising U.S. sales and their beneficial impact on incentives for R & D have been aided by the globalization of markets and longer profitable life spans for some drug specialties.

[10] T. R. Stauffer, "Discovery Risk, Profitability Performance, and Survival Risk in a Pharmaceutical Firm," *Regulation, Economics and Pharmaceutical Innovation*, ed. Joseph D. Cooper (Washington, D.C.: American University).

[11] David Schwartzman, *Innovation in the Pharmaceutical Industry* (Baltimore: Johns Hopkins University Press), 1976.

[12] David F. Saks, "The Resurgence in New Drug Activity," *Wertheim Industry Commentary* (February 7, 1979), p. 3.

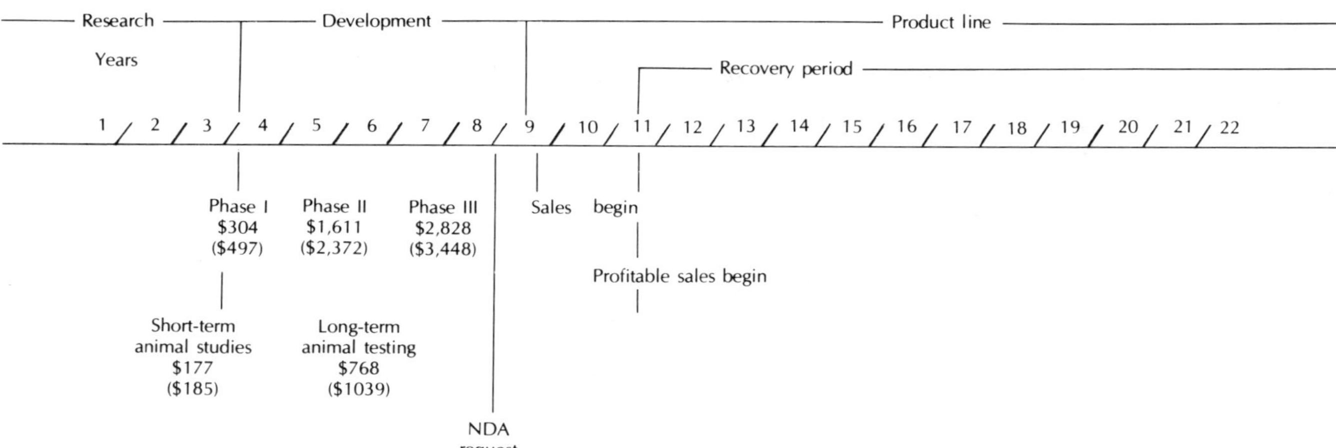

Figure 3-2. R & D time and cost for the average new chemical entity. All figures are expressed in thousands of 1976 dollars. (Those in parentheses represent an 8% capitalization of prior R & D expense.) [SOURCE: Modified from Harold A. Clymer, "The Economics of Drug Innovation," *The Development and Control of New Products,* eds. M. Pernarowski and M. Darrach (Vancouver: University of British Columbia) to reflect the cost of the average NCE that began to be tested in humans from 1963 to 1975. These figures are based on Ronald Hansen's study of 65 NCEs developed during that period of time. See Ronald W. Hansen, "The Pharmaceutical Development Process: Estimates of Current Development Costs and Times and the Effects of Regulatory Changes," Paper GPB 77-10 (Center for Research in Government Policy and Business of the Graduate School of Management, University of Rochester, revised July, 1978).]

Table 3-1. Major Prescription Branded Drugs

	Year of U.S. Introduction	*Annual Worldwide Sales[a] (millions)*	*Major Use*	*Company*
1977 introduction				
1. Valium	1963	$600	Tranquilizer	Hoffmann-La Roche
2. Aldomet	1963	350	Blood pressure	Merck
3. Garamycin	1968	240	Infection	Schering-Plough
4. Indocin	1965	200	Arthritis	Merck
5. Lasix	1966	200	Blood pressure	Hoechst
6. Inderal	1966	200	Blood pressure	American Home Products[b]
7. Vibramycin	1967	200	Infection	Pfizer
8. Keflex	1973	200	Infection	Eli Lilly
9. Ovral	1967	150	Birth control	American Home Products
10. Motrin	1974	150	Arthritis	Upjohn[b]
11. Keflin-N	1975	150	Infection	Eli Lilly
Recent introduction				
12. Tagamet	1977	500[c]	Ulcers	SmithKline
13. Clinoril	1978	250[c]	Arthritis	Merck
Future introduction				
14. Cefaclor	1979E	[d]	Infection	Eli Lilly
15. Dolobid	1981E	[d]	Pain reliever	Merck
16. Moducren	1981E	[d]	Blood pressure	Merck
17. Metramycin	1980E	[d]	Infection	Schering-Plough
18. Selacryn	1979E	[d]	Blood pressure	SmithKline
19. Auranofin	1982E	[d]	Arthritis	SmithKline
20. Captopril	1981E	[d]	Blood pressure	Squibb

SOURCE: David F. Saks, "The Resurgence in New Drug Activity," *Wertheim Industry Commentary* (February 7, 1979), p. 3. Used with permission.

[a] Wertheim estimate.

[b] U.S. and Canadian rights only.

[c] Potential. Actual sales in 1978 were about $280 million for Tagamet and $25 million for Clinoril.

[d] Worldwide sales could exceed $150 million in some cases and to some extent at the expense of other drugs on this list.

Table 3-2. R & D Expenditures

	Expenditures in 1977 (millions)	*Percentage Growth 1975–1977*
American Home Products	$ 66	18
Bristol-Myers	81	28
Eli Lilly	125	20
Merck	145	16
Pfizer	98	24
Schering-Plough	59	24
Searle	53	(−6)
SmithKline	62	18
Squibb	55	12
Sterling Drug	39	23
Syntax	28	33
Upjohn	102	31
Warner-Lambert	81	9

SOURCE: David F. Saks, "The Resurgence in New Drug Activity," *Wertheim Industry Commentary* (February 7, 1979), p. 8. Used with permission.

In looking at any new drug possibility, a number of organizational factors are considered beyond direct marketing and scientific strategies.[13]

- timing of the project in relation to other activities
- prestige and image value to the company
- effect on organizational esprit-de-corps
- impact of government and public opinion and other environmental factors
- alternative uses of scientific and other personnel in the event of a project failure
- moral compulsion to develop drugs of limited commercial value

FACTORS INFLUENCING R & D INCENTIVES

A variety of factors influence the way a company's objectives interact with its R & D incentives. Two of the most important factors are the

[13]Richard E. Faust, "Project Selection in the Pharmaceutical Industry," *Research Management*, Vol. 14 (1971).

knowledge base available for drug research and the cost of developing a new drug for the market, including the cost of complying with government regulations.

Diseases are puzzles that pharmaceutical scientists attempt to solve. Drug therapy is the use of chemicals to overcome or prevent undesirable conditions in the body. Some people have argued that the decline in the number of new chemical entities as well as current limitations on drug R & D arise from a depletion of the store of basic science. There are supporters and opponents of this "biological knowledge gap" thesis. If aspects of the puzzle for a particular drug or disease appear relatively unsolvable, companies will avoid the problem. Where breakthroughs appear likely and companies have the funds, they may do basic or fundamental research on the question. About 10% and 15% of industry spending has been for this type of research.

Experts on biomedical and pharmaceutical research have identified the following areas as most promising for fundamental research breakthroughs: neurobiology, immunology, molecular biology, cellular differentiation and cell membrane studies, and genetics.[14]

The ability of research breakthroughs to alter incentives for R & D applies not only to the drugs themselves but also to the way they are produced and/or delivered. For example, the Futures Group of Glastonbury, Connecticut, has suggested that breakthroughs in drug delivery systems such as alternatives to the familiar pill have a 75% likelihood of occurring in the next few years and that their promise could result in a rise of as much as 5% in overall R & D spending.[15] Likewise, breakthroughs in the use of recombinant DNA techniques to allow the production of drug therapies involving macromolecules would make a variety of new drug production possibilities more attractive.

Another cost item involved in developing a drug is compliance with required testing. Since 1962 new drugs marketed in the United States have been required to meet tests of efficacy and safety. The impact of the 1962 amendments to the federal Food, Drug, and Cosmetic Act of

[14]Lewis Thomas, "Biomedical Science and Human Health: The Long-range Prospect," *Daedalus* (Summer, 1977); Max Tishler and Robert G. Dankewalter, "Drug Research—Whence and Whither," *Progress in Drug Research*, ed. Ernest Jucker (Basel, Switzerland: Birkhauser, 1966).

[15]The Futures Group, Pharmaceutical PROSPECTS, "Research and Development Expenditures for Ethical Drugs" (Glastonbury, Conn.: The Futures Group, August, 1978), p. 13.

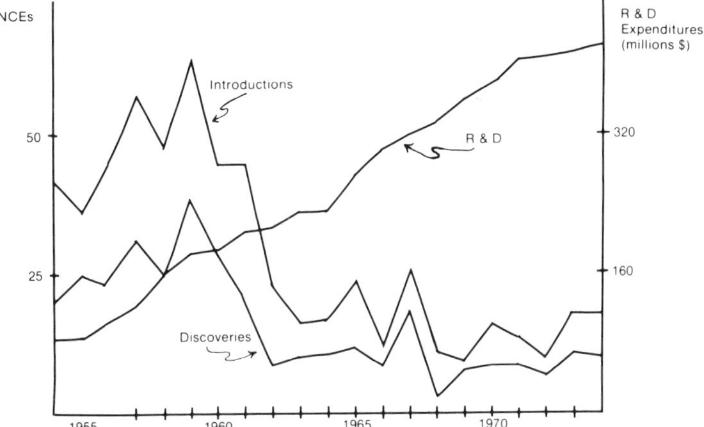

Figure 3-3. Introductions and discoveries of new chemical entities by domestic firms and constant 1958 dollar expenditures on pharmaceutical R & D, the United States, 1954–1974. [SOURCE: Henry G. Grabowski, John M. Vernon, and Lacy Glenn Thomas, "The Effects of Regulatory Policy on the Incentives to Innovate: An International Comparative Analysis" in *Impact of Public Policy on Drug Innovation and Pricing,* eds. Samuel A. Mitchell and Emery A. Link (Washington, D.C.: American University), p. 50. Used with permission.]

1938 has received extensive attention.[16] The situation prompting this concern is illustrated in Figure 3-3.

The introduction of NCEs is often used as a measure of innovation, despite important criticism of the utility of this measure. Figure 3-3 shows a marked decline in the number of NCEs introduced. Yet during the same period, R & D expenditures increased approximately fourfold.

[16]Samuel Peltzman, *Regulation of Pharmaceutical Innovation* (Washington, D.C.: American Enterprise Institute, 1974); Martin Neil Baily, "Research and Development Cost and Returns: The U.S. Pharmaceutical Industry," *Journal of Political Economy*, Vol. 80 (January-February, 1972), pp. 70–85; J. M. Jadrow, Jr., "The Economic Effects of the 1962 Drug Amendments," Unpublished Ph.D. Dissertation (University of Virginia, 1970); James M. Jondrow, "A Measure of the Monetary Benefits and Costs of the Regulation of Prescription Drug Effectiveness," Unpublished Ph.D. Dissertation (University of Virginia, 1972); Wardell and Lasagna, *op. cit.*; Henry Grabowski, John M. Vernon, and Lacy Glenn Thomas, "The Effects of Regulatory Policy on the Incentives to Innovate: An International Comparative Analysis," *Impact of Public Policy on Drug Innovation and Pricing*, eds. Samuel A. Mitchell and Emery A. Link (Washington, D.C.: American University, 1976), pp. 47–82; Schwartzman, *op cit.*; Nicholas A. Ashford, Stewart E. Butler, and Eric M. Zolt, "Regulation and Innovation in the Pharmaceutical Industry" (MIT Center for Policy Alternatives, July 1, 1977).

Studies generally agree that regulation has increased the cost of innovation and is partly responsible for the decline in NCEs. Henry Grabowski's analysis is one of the most recent and balanced studies. He compared the drug development processes of the United States with those of the United Kingdom, where safety and efficacy requirements are not as stringent.

> A principal finding that emerged from this analysis is that U.S. "productivity"—defined as the number of NCEs discovered and introduced in the United States per dollar R & D expenditure—declined by about sixfold between 1960–1961 and 1966–1970. The corresponding decrease in the United Kingdom was about threefold. Clearly, some worldwide phenomenon, which might be labeled a "depletion of research opportunities" seems to hold for pharmaceutical R & D. However, there is strong support for the hypothesis that an additional factor is at work in the U.S. industry. We contend that this additional factor, which has lowered U.S. productivity at a significantly more rapid rate, is the increased regulatory tightness resulting from the 1962 amendments. On the basis of a more sophisticated econometric analysis . . . we estimate that the 1962 amendments have roughly doubled the cost of a NCE.[17]

Costs have increased sixfold: about one-third of this increase can be attributed to the effects of more stringent regulations and the remaining two-thirds to a variety of factors.[18]

- relative shift of dollars from research to development (three major companies showed a 15% to 25% shift of budget from research to development in 10 years)
- shift of some research activity of multinational firms overseas
- concentration of R & D activity and innovation in the larger firms
- quest for epidemiologically more important drugs—those with larger markets
- diminution of some "me-too" research

To what extent regulation should be blamed or credited for the factors listed above is uncertain, but the ratio of one-third might apply here as well. In addition, there are some factors that have been

[17]Henry G. Grabowski, *Drug Regulation and Innovation: Empirical Evidence and Policy Options* (Washington, D.C.: American Enterprise Institute, 1975), p. 77.

[18]Grabowski, *op. cit.*; Lewis Sarrett, "FDA Regulations and Their Influence on Future Research and Development," *Research Management*, Vol. 17 (March, 1974), pp. 18–20.

important in elevating the cost of R & D, but they have received less attention.[19]

- development of more stringent scientific standards of acceptable evidence that, though more costly, probably would be used by drug companies even in the absence of government regulations
- greater concern for carcinogenic effects of drugs resulting in more conservative introduction by companies
- expanded prior testing to avoid consumer suits and liability hazards in the absence of regulation
- call by physicians for better tested drugs as a result of malpractice suits
- influence of the thalidomide incident even without the 1962 amendments

Despite those factors at work during the 1960s and 1970s, the peak in NCEs was reached in 1959. The decline in NCEs coincides with a decline in confidence in drug therapies and in the FDA. It is alleged that the 1962 amendments, rather than being a burden, actually provided a confidence rating or seal of government approval for new drugs. James Turner argues that it was the year *after* the passage of the amendments that the precipitous decline in the number of NCEs bottomed out and began to rise.[20]

Nicholas Ashford contended that the full impact of the 1962 amendments cannot be accurately gauged until these more subtle factors are considered and until the analysis is disaggregated to the therapeutic class of drug. Therapeutic class disaggregation is necessary, he asserted, because the classes represent different safety/efficacy tradeoffs, because they are affected differently by FDA actions, because they are in different stages of technological evolution, because they are administered differently by physicians, and because they are subject to different amounts of market competition.[21] Others have argued strongly that the long-term decline is closely related to the introduction of the 1962 amendments.

[19]Ashford *et al., op. cit.*

[20]James Turner, Testimony to the U.S. Senate Select Committee on Small Business, *Hearings on Competitive Problems in the Drug Industry*, 92nd Congress (Washington, D.C.: U.S. Government Printing Office, 1974). See also "Highlights of the Discussion," Chapter 1.

[21]Ashford *et al., op. cit.*

COMPANY RESPONSES TO RAISED OR LOWERED R & D COSTS

Thus far, company responses to rising R & D costs have included:

- raising R & D expenditures, particularly where sales are increasing
- diminishing R & D expenditures within firms near the margin of successful return on drugs in smaller or more competitive markets
- diversifying to compensate for a poor rate of return on research investment and to utilize the larger profits from prior research investment
- shifting effort overseas
- merger activities
- licensing and technology transfer
- strengthening ties with academic and government research efforts
- changing the structure of R & D to emphasize more development and less research and to concentrate on drugs for larger markets

If costs were lowered as a result of a change in regulatory practices, firms would have all of the above options plus the choice of raising profits, modernizing plants and equipment, lowering prices, or some combination thereof.

HEALTH COSTS AND BENEFITS OF THE REGULATIONS

Cost/benefit analyses of the amendments implicitly or explicitly deal with health outcomes. Two studies illustrating the approach and the results reach divergent conclusions. James Jondrow estimated a favorable benefit/cost ratio for the 1962 amendments of 2.24 based on the decrease in sales of "ineffective" drugs as measured by the National Academy of Sciences review of drug efficacy.[22]

Using the economic notion of "consumer surplus," Samuel Peltzman estimated that the amendments resulted in an annual loss of $300 million to $400 million in benefits from the reduced flow of new drugs, a gain of under $100 million from reduced waste on purchases of ineffective drugs, and a loss of $50 million from reduced competition from new drugs. This represents a net annual loss of about $350 million, or about 6% of total drug sales.[23]

[22]Jondrow, *op. cit.*

[23]Peltzman, *op. cit.*, pp. 170–172.

Jondrow's study has been criticized for the measures of ineffective drugs he used,[24] while Peltzman's estimates have been criticized for attributing all of the increase in cost to the amendments, for attributing more conscious choice to consumers than commonly occurs in drug therapy markets, and for other technical issues.[25]

Industry spokespeople have argued that the amendments have made companies less able and willing to pursue "me-too" drugs of little therapeutic value.[26] Former FDA Commissioner Alexander Schmidt used a similar type of argument to defend the amendments. Schmidt contended that the amendments reduced significantly the number of drugs of little or no therapeutic value while having little impact on therapeutically important drugs. Figure 3-4 shows the introduction of NCEs and classifies new drugs according to therapeutic gain as rated by the FDA. Schmidt argued that the number of therapeutically important new drugs has remained fairly constant at about five to seven a year. Likewise, drugs of most therapeutic gain have remained at about the same level. It is drugs of little therapeutic gain that were most affected in relation to the pre-amendment period.[27]

The FDA has ranked drugs four different times for the period 1950 through 1973; Grabowski argued that the divergence among these four lists is too great to make them credible, while Ashford argued that, except for the first ranking, they are consistent. Schmidt's argument was not based on the earliest ranking.[28] Ratings of therapeutic importance continue to raise troublesome questions about the effects of drug R & D. Schmidt's earlier figures tend to be supported by FDA ratings of drugs approved for marketing from October, 1975, through June, 1978: of the 72 new molecular entities introduced, 9 represent important therapeutic gains, 20 represent modest therapeutic gains, while 43 were judged to have little or no therapeutic gain.[29] On the other hand, the Pharmaceutical Manufacturers Association argued that some drugs not listed as therapeutic

[24]Grabowski, *op. cit.*, p. 66.

[25]*Ibid*, pp. 70–74, and Turner, *op. cit.*

[26]Sarrett, *op. cit.*

[27]Alexander Schmidt, Testimony to the U.S. Senate Subcommittee on Health of the Committee on Labor and Public Welfare, *Hearings on Legislation Amending the Public Health Service Act and the Federal Food, Drug, and Cosmetic Act*, 93rd Congress (Washington, D.C.: U.S. Government Printing Office, 1974), pp. 3077–3103.

[28]Grabowski, *op. cit.*, and Ashford *et al.*, *op. cit.*

[29]FDA Ratings of New Drugs," *Consumer Reports*, Vol. 43, No. 10 (October, 1978), pp. 578–581.

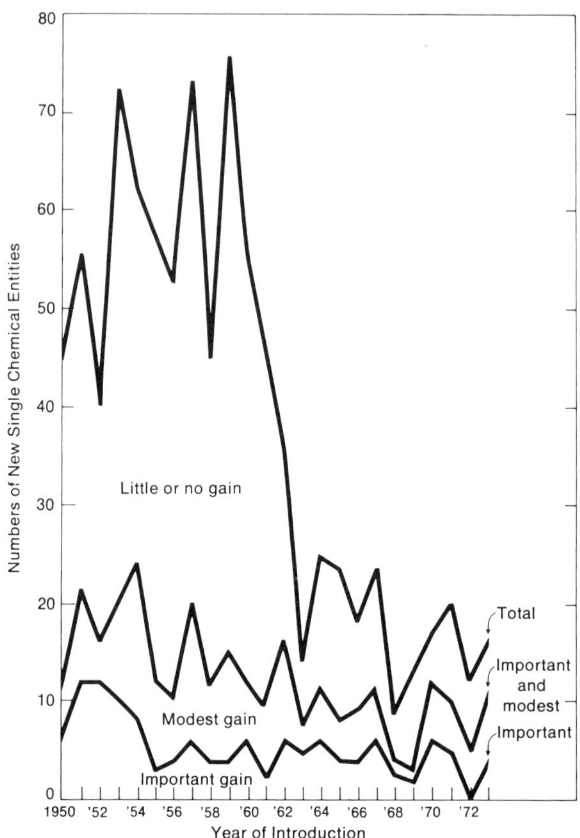

Figure 3-4. FDA classification of annual new drug approvals by degree of therapeutic importance, 1950–1973. [SOURCE: Henry G. Grabowski, *Drug Regulation and Innovation: Empirical Evidence and Policy Options,* based on data from testimony of Alexander Schmidt to U.S. Senate Subcommittee on Health of the Committee on Labor and Public Welfare, *Hearings on Legislation Amending the Public Health Service Act and the Federal Food, Drug, and Cosmetic Act,* 93rd Congress (Washington, D.C.: American Enterprise Institute), p. 18. Copyright 1976 American Enterprise Institute. Reprinted with permission.]

gains by the FDA actually represent improvements because of altered side effects for some patients and because the therapeutic gains of some drugs for secondary indications are often discovered only after marketing.[30]

[30]C. Joseph Steter, Letter to *Consumer Reports* in Response to "FDA Ratings of New Drugs" (Washington, D.C.: Pharmaceutical Manufacturers Association).

By delaying the testing of drugs on humans, the higher costs and more stringent regulations may have had an additional subtle effect on innovation because of a decrease in the opportunity for serendipitous observations during human testing. For example, because of his observations made while using dopamine to treat other conditions, pharmacologist Leon Goldberg has added dopamine to the therapies useful in treating shock.[31] Although there is some argument over the degree to which serendipity is still a major factor in drug discovery, it has been said to account for as much as one-half of all new drugs and new uses of existing drugs. Undoubtedly, however, serendipity has been hindered by the decrease in testing, for which the regulations are partly responsible.

In recent years, the increased costs brought about in part by federal regulations have discouraged some small firms and some larger firms from doing research and have led others to concentrate on developing drugs discovered elsewhere. However, the major research-oriented companies have been able to bear the higher costs. There does appear to be greater concentration of innovation as a result of the cost increases,[32] which may eventually result in greater concentration in sales.

Increasing costs have shifted incentives toward more therapeutically important drugs for epidemiologically more important diseases. While the majority of these drugs are not of significant therapeutic gain, this shift in attention has led to great success for companies with "jackpot" drugs. It has also made "orphan" drugs, those of limited commercial value, less likely to be sought or developed.

Most of the published academic data deal with the 1960s and early 1970s, a period in which one observer noted, "The incentive for investment has already been substantially weakened. The financial community has already taken note of these developments. Very few industrial analysts now look upon the drug industry with favor, or —as they once did—as a growth industry."[33] This situation may have changed since 1976, according to one investment analyst. Saks notes, "After several years of quiescence, a number of major new drugs have burst upon the scene, generating both rapid success and growing excitement in and around the drug industry. Accounting for this phenomenon are two basic factors that appear likely to sustain a high

[31]Leon I. Goldberg, "Creativity in New Drug Development: An Academic Challenge," *Perspectives in Biology and Medicine* (Winter, 1978), pp. 188–195.

[32]Grabowski, *op. cit.*

[33]Hansen, *op. cit.*, p. 3.

level of interest in new drug activity for some time to come."[34] The two factors are (1) marked improvement in the regulatory environment from the FDA and (2) a reorientation of drug research toward new disease categories that promise to yield a series of new and improved remedies whose success is to a greater extent incremental rather than at the expense of existing sales.

Saks ascribed the changes at the FDA to pressures from Congress, the medical community, and consumer groups. Nelson Schneider, a pharmaceutical analyst at E. F. Hutton, confirmed this impression and suggested that the existence of the proposed Drug Regulation Reform Bill and the pressures around it were the cause of the change at the FDA. While pharmaceutical industry personnel dispute the notion that regulatory burdens have been eased, if Schneider's perception is correct, the proposed drug regulation bill has already favorably affected the incentives for R & D.

There are several provisions in the proposed Drug Regulation Reform Bill that might affect R & D incentives, including release of safety and efficacy data for use after 5 years, postmarketing surveillance of new drugs, requirement of a formalized IND approval system, including a plan for investigation, protocols, and so forth, greater public participation in the drug approval process, export of unapproved drugs, annual drug experience assessment report, and research activities at the proposed National Center for Drug Science.

The disagreement between investment analysts and industry spokespeople over the proposed drug regulation bill shows the difficulty of pointing to a specific action and attaching consequences to it. The problem is further illustrated by the FDA's analysis of the economic impact of the bill[35] and the Pharmaceutical Manufacturers Association's (PMA) response to it. Attention here will focus on the provisions that would allow immediate release of safety and efficacy data for the purpose of public participation in the drug approval process and the use of the data by another company in registering its drug under the innovator's monograph.

The release of safety and efficacy data would make it easier for other companies to copy the discoveries made by innovating firms by producing exact copies of generic drugs, or drugs similar to patented drugs. The proposed bill prohibits use of such data in the United States for drug approval purposes for 5 years, and in the process gives

[34] Saks, *op. cit.*

[35] Fay Dworkin, "An Analysis of the Economic Impact of the Drug Regulation Reform Act of 1978," Office of Planning and Evaluation, FDA (November, 1978).

an advantage to foreign producers who have access to and can use the data in their countries' approval process. The FDA estimates that from $368 to $1,444 million of sales of U.S. products would be vulnerable to sales by foreign companies as a result of this provision. Using a figure in the lower part of this range—$599 million lost to foreign competition—and assuming present ratios of R & D to sales, the FDA forecast implies a decrease in R & D spending of $54 million. Among companies competing for domestic sales of generic drugs, the release of this data would put the nonresearch intensive firms in a comparatively better position and lead to a shift in sales to such companies. However, because of the 5-year ban, this impact would be slight, leading at most to a decrease in R & D expenditures of $1 million.[36]

The PMA's response is that the $54 million figure is too low. Added to already declining R & D-to-sales ratios for some companies, foreign competition will accelerate the decline, it claims. Also, the loss of approximately 6% of R & D would have a disproportionate effect on R & D productivity because of the substantial fixed costs of R & D. The shift of sales to nonresearch intensive firms would result in decreased innovation of important drugs rather than of new formulations. Many potential drugs are near or below the estimated annual global sales of $10 to $12 million; increased competition would make this figure even more difficult to achieve.

Both the FDA and the PMA agree, however, that there is insufficient information to assess economic impact accurately, much less to gauge the effect of changes in R & D incentives on the kinds of new drugs developed.

[36] *Ibid.*

HIGHLIGHTS OF THE DISCUSSION

A review of the average costs of discovering and developing a new chemical entity (see Table 3-3) led to disagreement about the amount and type of R & D necessary and the impact of regulations on R & D.

William Comanor, director of the Bureau of Economics of the Federal Trade Commission, felt that the literature on the discovery and development of NCEs offers a misleading picture of government policy and does not focus adequately on the real issues involved. He argued against assuming necessarily that research should grow as quickly and extensively as possible, pointing out that research could become too large and develop more drugs of lower overall therapeutic gain if a simple approach to speeding up testing is taken. He suggested that we think in terms of "optimum" rather than "maximum" innovation: the greatest amount of therapeutic gain rather than the largest number of new drugs on the market.

Comanor also noted two other problems: (1) rapid product development and price competition give rise to a different type of market structure; and (2) physicians cannot absorb information on an excessive number of new drugs.

Hubert Peltier, senior vice president for research and development for Merck, Sharp & Dohme Laboratories, responded to Comanor by noting that many questions remain unanswered. To restrict research would limit opportunities for finding new therapeutic agents for diseases such as arthritis for which there are still no cures. He also commented that it would be arbitrary for the government to set up disincentives for taking risks to develop drugs. There is a need, and a public perception of a need, for new drugs, many of which have small markets. These require special incentives for discovery and development.

Leon Goldberg, professor of pharmacology and medicine at the University of Chicago, outlined what is necessary to make a drug discovery and the implications this process has for R & D. Drugs are found not only through planning but also by coincidence, he explained. If researchers are prevented from doing experiments, we will lose knowledge about the substance under investigation, about the possibility of side effects and interactions with other drugs, and about unexpected consequences of the drug under study. Such findings often take a long time to recognize and understand. He also

Table 3-3. Costs of Discovering and Developing a New Chemical Entity (NCE)

	R & D Costs (millions)	*Percentage of Total R & D Costs*[a]
Discovery		
Average cost per successful NCE, including cost of failures	$16	30%
8% capitalization	14	25
Discovery subtotal	(30)	
Development		
Average cost per successful NCE	6	11
Cost for the seven compounds that are rejected	11	20
8% capitalization	7	13
Development subtotal	(24)	
Total R & D costs for the average NCE	$54	100%

SOURCE: Ronald W. Hansen, "The Pharmaceutical Development Process: Estimates of Current Development Costs and Times and the Effects of Regulatory Changes," Paper GPB 77-10 (Center for Research in Government Policy and Business, Graduate School of Management, University of Rochester, revised July, 1978).
[a]Figures do not total due to rounding.

remarked that there is considerable difficulty in applying findings from animal studies to humans.

Goldberg also noted that the real question is how much regulation is really necessary. People with legal and economic training, he said, do not have the same background as medical doctors or pharmaceutical experts for understanding incentives and disincentives for research. Presently, there are few rewards for taking a chance in drug R & D. Referring to decreased budgets, fewer research physicians, ethical problems, and other factors, Goldberg commented that we are "on the descending limb of creativity."

An important trend in drug R & D, Goldberg added, is the change of companies from family-type efforts to corporate entities. Family companies showed greater concern for creative research and often had close, enduring relationships with investigators. In general, large companies are concerned with quantity and profit and tend to lack the sense of creativity demonstrated by family companies.

One participant outlined the effects the then-pending Drug Regulation Reform Act of 1979 may have on drug R & D and argued that it would, on the whole, have a positive impact because it would cut the

I. By providing greater predictability to the approval process:
   A. FDA required to establish guidelines for drug testing.
   B. FDA required to respond to drug companies that seek advice regarding their testing plans, protocols, and methods as well as the acceptability of their results.
   C. Procedure established for resolving scientific disputes between drug companies and the FDA.

II. By placing less of an "all-or-nothing" burden for proof on the FDA:
   A. FDA can allow limited distribution of a drug whose safety and efficacy cannot otherwise be determined.
   B. Patients will be required to give their informed consent where FDA finds that the drug poses a serious risk.
   C. FDA may subject new drugs to postmarket surveillance.
   D. FDA can allow "breakthrough drugs"—lifesaving drugs with unique therapeutic advantages—to be available for seriously ill patients who have no therapeutic alternatives if the drug appears effective even though testing is not complete.
   E. Public participation is encouraged by allowing comment at all proceedings and providing funding for participation in some.

Figure 3-5. Potential effects of the drug regulation reform act of 1979 on incentives for drug R & D.

time and cost involved in R & D. The bill would consolidate industry guidelines and decrease the uncertainty surrounding the FDA's acceptance of research results. It would provide the FDA with stricter guidelines, establish a procedure for resolving scientific disputes, and include a breakthrough provision to make drugs under testing available to those who are very ill. Overall, the bill would make drug approval more flexible. These and other aspects of the bill that could affect incentives for drug R & D are identified in Figure 3-5.

Several other concerns were also expressed:

1. One participant claimed that although legislation would provide for stability and consistency over time, we could possibly achieve the same results through regulations instead of a bill, particularly since the FDA has a marked ability to restrict the marketing of drugs now. This contention was countered with the argument that new regulations would only further complicate an already overloaded method of drug regulation.

2. More information is needed about who approves or rejects a particular drug. Such persons are not accountable to the public at the present time, and increased public awareness and reviewer accountability could improve the current system.

3. Regarding disclosure, some concern was voiced over the privacy of research data. It was pointed out, however, that the bill would not require publication of raw data and would thus protect the innovator

from competitors. A question was also raised about the effect of increased disclosure on the quality of drugs.

4. Orphan drugs—those for which there is not a large market—were discussed in connection with diversification in drug R & D. Peltier noted that most areas of drug research are covered today and that drug researchers have the interest and willingness but not the leads necessary to make significant breakthroughs on orphan drugs.

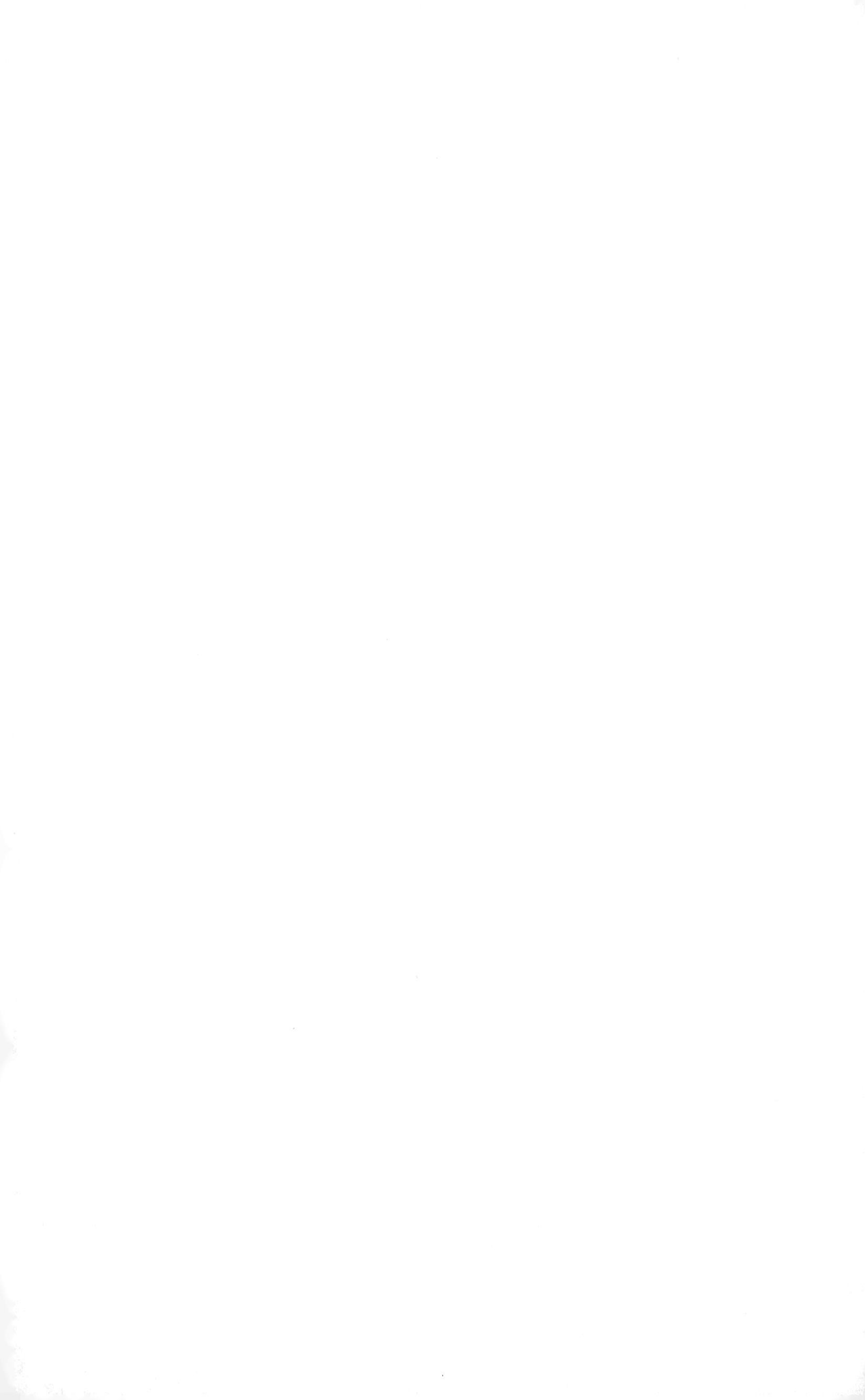

4

National Health Insurance: What Effect on Pharmaceutical R & D?

Escalating costs of health care have recently generated mounting public demand for some form of national health insurance. Such protection, which would aid patients in meeting the costs of physicians' services, hospital care, and prescription drugs, has been advocated for three reasons. First, many lower-income patients have no health insurance; Medicaid coverage is often insufficient and is not uniformly administered from state to state. Second, those who do have health insurance are often unprotected against catastrophic illnesses. Third, current health insurance programs are said to perpetuate inefficient, high-cost health care and discourage the practice of preventative medicine.[1]

Several national health insurance (NHI) proposals have been introduced in Congress. Although there are major differences between the plans, most contain proposals for coverage of prescription drugs.[2]

While prescription drugs represent only about one-tenth of national health care costs, they contribute more significantly to health care outcomes than more costly therapies.[3] Industry has been the major source of new drug development for the past three decades. Since industry finances its research out of its profits, the impact of

[1] Walter J. Campbell, "The Emerging Health Care Environment: Selected Issues," in *The Pharmaceutical Industry*, ed. Cotton M. Lindsay (New York: John Wiley & Sons, 1978), pp. 119–140.

[2] Milton Silverman and Mia Lydecker, *Drug Coverage Under National Health Insurance: The Policy Options* (Washington, D.C.: National Center for Health Services Research, 1978), pp. 58–61.

[3] Victor Fuchs, *Who Shall Live? Health, Economics and Social Choice* (New York: Basic Books, 1974), pp. 105–127.

national health insurance on doctor and hospital visits, on prescribing practices, and on the price of drugs is likely to affect the level and direction of industry research.

THE PHARMACEUTICAL R & D PROCESS

In 1977 an estimated $5,526 million was spent in the United States on health-related R & D. Of this, $1,625 million was spent by industry, primarily by pharmaceutical companies. The federal government spent $3,351 million on research, primarily conducted at the National Institutes of Health (NIH).[4] Figure 4-1 identifies the trends in this spending from 1968 through 1977.

Except for research conducted at various NIH institutes, federal drug R & D efforts are often the by-products of other programs. A major summary of federal government activity in drug R & D prepared in 1975 by Edward Burger for the Office of the Science Advisor to the President stated:

> Government (federal) R & D activities which contribute to the evolution of new and better medicines evolved typically and primarily from scientific curiosity about physiological and biochemical processes and mechanisms of diseases—not from concerted attempts at drug development. While this underlying feature remains predominant, a number of programs specifically aimed at new and better drugs have been mounted by the government—especially by NIH.[5]

The directions of and incentives for government-sponsored research differ from the motivations and objectives of pharmaceutical industry research. Scientific interest and medical importance rather than size of the prospective profit are the driving factors of government-sponsored research. Hence, the patentability of new chemicals and uses is usually of secondary importance. The government pays far more attention to basic biological research on the molecular and cellular basis of disease than does industry. The government also devotes significant attention to diseases affecting small populations.

[4]"Basic Data Relating to the National Institutes of Health," *NIH Factbook* (Washington, D.C.: Government Printing Office, March, 1978), p. 4.

[5]Edward J. Burger, "The Current Role of the Federal Government in Drug Related R & D: What Is It and What Should It Be?" *Impact of Public Policy on Drug Innovation and Pricing*, eds. Samuel A. Mitchell and Emery A. Link (Washington, D.C.: The American University, 1976), p. 409.

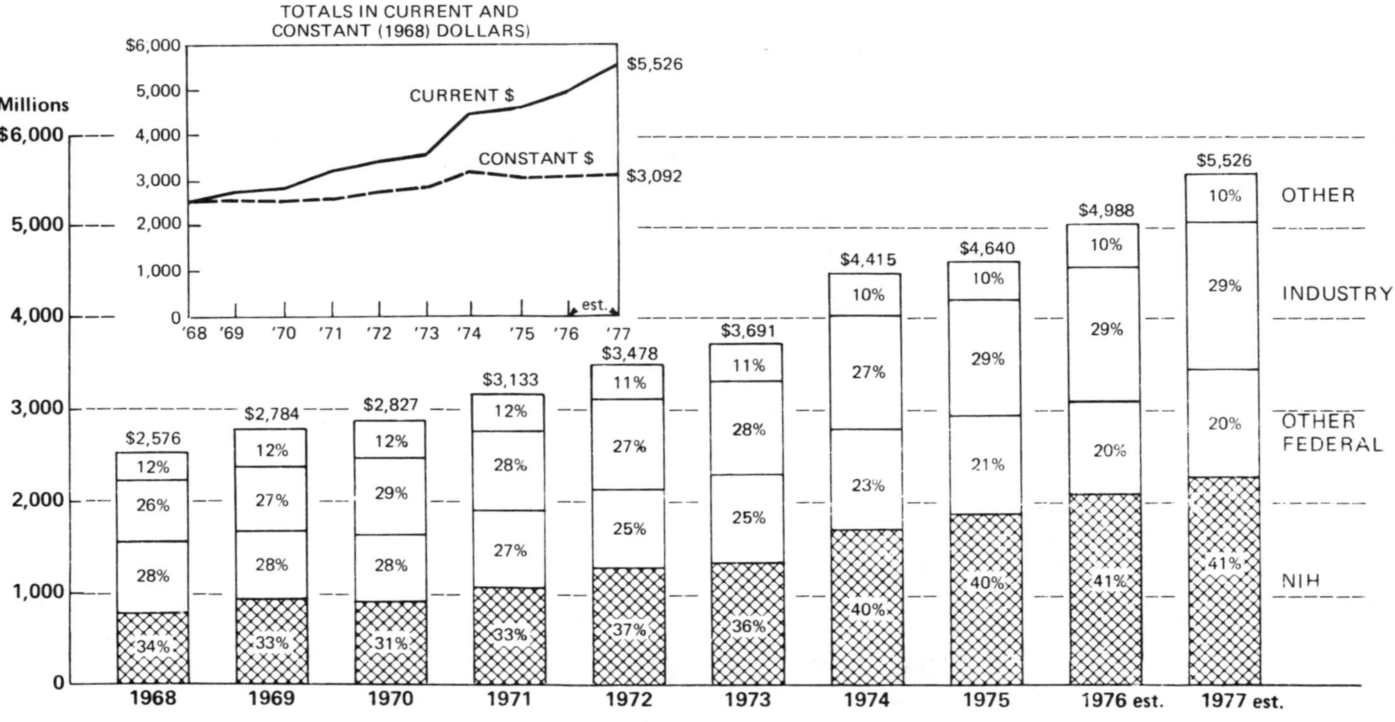

Figure 4-1. National support for health R & D by source, 1968–1977. (Dollars in millions. Constant dollars based on revised biomedical R & D deflator—over $2,244 million in 1977, including $1,436 grants, $394 contracts, $248 intramural research, etc.) [SOURCE: "Basic Data Relating to the National Institutes of Health," *NIH Factbook* (Washington, D.C.: Government Printing Office, March 1978), p. 4.]

With respect to drug R & D, each institute of the NIH has a specific set of objectives. The National Cancer Institute researches anticancer drugs. Drug therapies for lowering blood lipids, preventing coronary artery disease, and treating hypertension and cardiac arrythmias are major interests of the National Heart and Lung Institute. Development of more effective contraceptives as well as drugs for chemotherapy of pediatric cancers are under investigation at the National Institute of Child Health and Human Development. Major research interests at the National Institute of Dental Research include drugs effective against caries and for use as adjuncts to oral surgery. The National Institute of Neurological Diseases and Stroke played a major role in the discovery and development of levodopa for Parkinson's disease; institute researchers are also studying drugs for use in paralysis and other neurological disorders. At the National Institute of General Medical Sciences, a pharmacology-toxicology program seeks more effective methods of discovering and developing new therapeutic agents.

Within their respective fields of interest, these institutes evaluate newly marketed drugs to confirm their therapeutic usefulness. New drugs are compared to established drugs to determine their relative efficacy, and tests are conducted to find new indications for existing drugs. Mechanisms of drug action attract far more attention than is usual in industry.[6]

In 1975 (the most recent year for which complete pharmaceutical data are available), R & D expenditures by the pharmaceutical industry were $1,000 million, or 76% of all industry health R & D and 22% of health R & D from all sources. Unlike government-sponsored research facilities, pharmaceutical companies must be concerned with profits in order to generate sufficient resources to support research. Resources for R & D are usually expressed as a percentage of sales. Figure 4-2 indicates the distribution of sales dollars by the average U.S. pharmaceutical manufacturer in the early to mid-1960s.

The precise percentage of R & D to sales varies depending on the source consulted. Silverman and Lee use 8% for the years 1970 to 1974. The Pharmaceutical Manufacturers Association's (PMA) estimate for its member firms is from 11% to 12%. In 1976 other figures for the industry were 7.6%, while the National Science Foundation (NSF), reporting on drugs and medicines, placed the figure at 7.5%. When considering the potential impact of national health insurance,

[6] *Ibid.*, pp. 394–403.

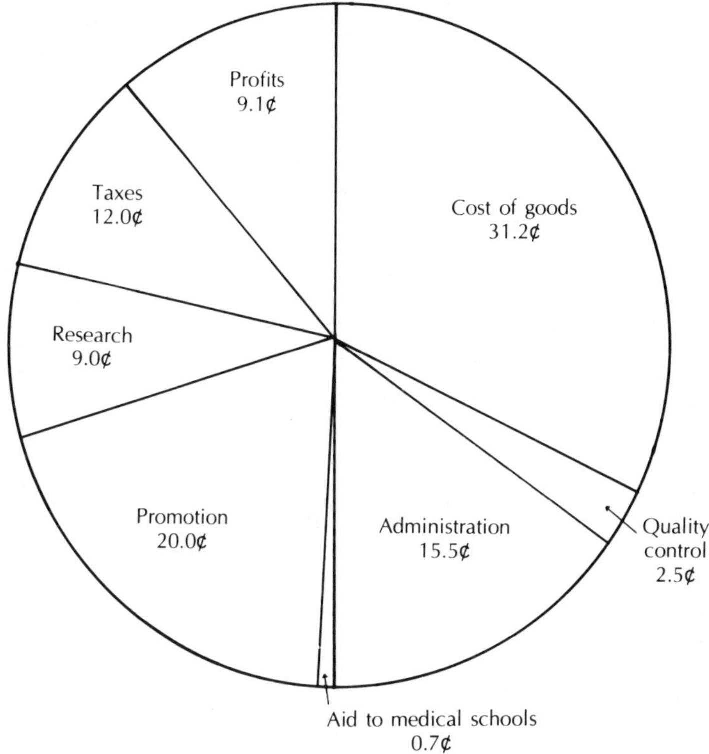

Figure 4-2. Distribution of pharmaceutical manufacturers' sales dollars. [SOURCE: Milton Silverman and Philip R. Lee, *Pills, Profits and Politics* (Los Angeles: University of California Press), p. 29. Reprinted by permission of the University of California Press. Information derived from extrapolation of data in U.S. Department of Health, Education, and Welfare Task Force on Prescription Drugs, *The Drug Makers and the Drug Distributors* (Washington, D.C.: Government Printing Office, 1968), p. 13.]

the important factor is that R & D has been a fairly stable percentage of sales for most companies.

In 1972 the 21 largest pharmaceutical companies had sales that accounted for 75.6% of the market. Table 4-1 lists these companies and the degree of change in their relative positions between 1962 and 1972.

While the aggregate picture of the industry suggests competition, the top four firms account in most instances for 50% to 60% of sales within specific product categories. This is so because the necessary expertise and production techniques vary dramatically across product

Table 4-1. Firm Turnover for the Leading 21 Firms in the Ethical Pharmaceutical Industry, 1962–1972

Company	*Market Share of Hospital and Drugstore Sales (percent of industry total)*		*Rank in Terms of Market Share*		*Change in Rank Between 1962 and 1972*
	1962	*1972*	*1962*	*1972*	
Lilly	7.2	7.9	1	1	0
Hoffmann-La Roche	4.0	7.5	10	2	+ 8
American Home Products	6.1	6.6	3	3	0
Merck	4.9	6.0	6	4	+ 2
Bristol-Myers	3.4	4.2	13	5	+ 8
Abbott	3.9	3.7	11	6	+ 5
Pfizer	3.8	3.6	12	7	+ 5
Ciba-Geigy	4.2	3.6	8	8	0
Upjohn	5.8	3.5	4	9	− 5
Squibb	4.1	3.4	9	10	− 1
SmithKline	6.3	3.3	2	11	− 9
Johnson & Johnson	1.3	2.7	21	12	+ 9
Schering-Plough	2.4	2.7	15	13	+ 2
Parke-Davis[a]	4.6	2.7	7	14	− 7
Searle	2.2	2.5	17	15	+ 2
Lederle	5.3	2.3	5	16	−11
Sandoz-Wander	1.6	2.0	19	17	+ 2
Robins	1.9	2.0	18	18	0
Sterling	2.4	1.9	16	19	− 3
Burroughs Wellcome	1.4	1.8	20	20	0
Warner-Lambert[a]	2.6	1.7	14	21	− 7
Average absolute change in rank between 1962 and 1972					4.1[b]

SOURCE: D. Cocks, "Production Innovation and the Dynamic Elements of Competition in the Ethical Pharmaceutical Industry," *Drug Development and Marketing,* ed. Robert B. Helms (Washington, D.C.: American Enterprise Institute for Public Policy Research), p. 241, copyright 1976 American Enterprise Institute. Used with permission.

[a] Parke-Davis was merged with Warner-Lambert in late 1970; rank and market shares computed as if firms had not merged. Market share of the combined firm in 1972 was 4.4 %, or fifth in rank.

[b] Computed with Parke-Davis and Warner-Lambert changes based on their ranks as if they had not merged.

lines and because one class of drug such as an antibiotic cannot be substituted for another such as an antihypertensive.

Drug types are commonly distinguished according to a product's use or therapeutic class. Table 4-2 details the major product classes, their ranks and percentage shares, sales, number of companies indicating sales, and the rank and percentage shares of applied R & D expenditures for 1974. By 1978 the anti-infective product class was receiving the greatest expenditures while the relative positions of the rest remained the same.

Figure 3-1 depicts the time frame within which companies operate in deciding, developing, and marketing a drug—25 years is the average, although longer approval periods and changes in the length of the period of legal monopoly from patent rights would change this. Table 4-3 gives the functional distribution of U.S. R & D expenditures in the industry for 1977.

For purposes of analyzing research directions, research activities may be conveniently broken down into four areas. Basic research is oriented toward the acquisition of new knowledge; it may or may not be directed at a specific clinical application. Applied research has as its objective the identification of compounds that will be clinically useful. Development research is concerned with development of dosage forms, modification of synthetic processes, and other activities directed toward bringing the product to the marketplace. Finally, defensive research is conducted to protect or advance the market position of existing product lines. This area of research includes Phase IV postmarketing surveillance and other studies required by the federal government to keep products on the market.

Basic or exploratory research is the key to the discovery of new pharmaceutical products. Estimates of basic research in industry vary from 10% to 20% of the total R & D effort. Unlike federally sponsored research, industrial research is decentralized; each firm directs its research programs according to its own objectives and motivations.

Of paramount concern to industrial research planners is probability of achieving project objectives. This is a function of many variables including the cost in time and dollars of achieving the objective. Obviously a firm will hesitate to commit time and money to a project if there is little or no probability of recouping investments. For this reason, the patentability or exclusivity of anticipated discoveries is a threshold consideration. If the company does not have a suitable pool of research talent from which to draw, another consideration is the cost of securing the personnel and resources needed to carry out the project. However, even if the project is not completed, it may serve as a springboard for future research activities.

Table 4-2. Product Classes, Selected Data

Rank	*Sales (in millions)*	*Percentage of Sales*	*Number of Companies Indicating Sales*	*Rank: Applied R & D Expenditures*[a]	*Percentage Share: Applied R & D Dollar*
1. Central nervous system	1,395.9	26.5	38	1	18.5
2. Anti-infectives	834.3	15.9	31	2	17.8
3. Neoplasms and endocrine system and metabolic disease	531.3	10.1	27	4	14.0
4. Digestives and genitourinary	519.9	9.9	38	5	6.2
5. Cardiovasculars	479.6	9.1	31	3	15.1
6. Vitamins and nutrients	457.4	8.7	32	9	2.1
7. Respiratory system	335.9	6.4	33	6	4.8
8. Dermatologicals	178.5	3.4	30	8	3.5
9. Biologicals	141.5	2.7	13	7	4.5
10. Diagnostic agents	113.5	2.1	14	—	—
11. Other	273.0	5.2	23		6.1
Veterinary preparations					6.9
Veterinary biologicals					.5

SOURCE: Pharmaceutical Manufacturers Association, *Annual Survey Report, 1974–1975* (Washington, D.C.: PMA, 1976), and *Research and Development in the Pharmaceutical Industry* (Washington, D.C.: PMA), p. 31. Used with permission.

[a]Based only on those PMA members reporting data.

Table 4-3. Distribution of U.S. R & D Expenditures for Ethical Pharmaceuticals, by Function, 1977

Function	*Percentage of Total*
Biological screening and pharmacological testing	18.7
Clinical evaluation: Phases I, II, III	17.8
Synthesis and extraction	17.2
Pharmaceutical dosage formulation and stability testing	9.7
Toxicology and safety testing	9.2
Process development for manufacturing and quality control	8.8
Clinical evaluation: Phase IV	4.7
Regulatory, IND and NDA preparation, submission, and processing	3.3
Bioavailability studies	2.3
Other	8.3
Total	100.0

SOURCE: Pharmaceutical Manufacturers Association, *Annual Survey: Ethical Pharmaceutical Industry Operations, 1977–1978* (Washington, D.C.: PMA), p. 24. Used with permission.

Marketing aspects also figure prominently in industrial research decisionmaking. Research planners consider whether there is a need for a particular product, whether a competitor is already meeting that need, and whether competing products are under development. In short, it must be decided whether a product under development can capture a share of the market large enough to justify R & D expenditures. Intangible factors such as the impact of governmental, environmental, and public opinion pressures, prestige and image value to the company, and timing in relation to other marketing and research activities are also aspects that must be considered.[7]

There is an ongoing debate over the merits of "me-too" (molecular modification) research versus "breakthrough" research. Drug industry spokespeople often claim that the burdens of the drug regulatory process have made it economically unfeasible to develop drugs with few advantages over existing products. However, me-too research can yield financial returns when molecular modification produces a drug that offers greater patient convenience, lower incidence of side effects, and a more effective mode of action. In fact, a recent article in

[7]Richard E. Faust, "Project Selection in the Pharmaceutical Industry," *Research Management* 14 (1971), p. 46.

Consumer Reports indicates that me-too research is widely conducted. In October, 1978, *Consumer Reports* published FDA ratings of products approved for marketing from October, 1975, through June, 1978. Only 9 represented modest therapeutic gains while 43 were rated by the FDA as representing little or no therapeutic gain. Of the remaining 148 drugs approved for marketing during that time, over 100 were me-too items.[8]

Another important issue shaping the future of pharmaceutical R & D is diversification. Continued investment in R & D is a function of anticipated return in relation to other investment opportunities: 12% return is a figure often cited as sufficient to justify reinvestment in innovation. In recent years, however, several companies have reduced their research activities and moved to diversify. In some cases, companies have moved into areas related to their existing research, bioengineering, and quality control capabilities. For example, Sandoz has moved into seeds, and Hoffmann-La Roche has established a diagnostics division and acquired a clinical laboratory subsidiary. Other firms have established entirely different product lines: Warner-Lambert operates businesses producing bakery products, optical goods, and other consumer products.

INTERACTION OF DRUG USE PATTERNS WITH NHI

A recent report prepared for the National Center for Health Services Research states:

> Among all forms of medical therapy, drug therapy is probably the most widely applied. In about 45% of all office visits, the physician prescribes or recommends the use of one or more drug products. For inpatients, it appears that an average of one prescription is written for each day of hospitalization, or about eight prescriptions for a typical hospital stay. Whether all these drugs, inpatient or outpatient, are rationally prescribed has been questioned. Whether all or even most of these drug orders are necessary is also a matter of concern. Some authorities have testified that as many as 25% of all prescriptions are unnecessary or call for a drug whose efficacy has never been demonstrated.
>
> Until recently, the use of prescription drugs in the United States as in most industrialized nations, has continued to climb year after year. For out-of-hospital drugs dispensed by community pharmacies alone, the number of prescriptions rose from approximately 363 million in 1950

[8]"FDA Ratings of New Drugs," *Consumer Reports*, Vol. 43, No. 10 (October, 1978), pp. 578–581.

and 634 million in 1960, and 1.2 billion in 1970. At the retail level, these products represented expenditures of about $736 million in 1950, $2 billion in 1960, and $4.8 billion in 1970. In 1974 and 1975, however, the total number of prescriptions showed little or no rise, although total expenditures for the products continued to increase. . . .

Prescription drug expenditures will probably continue to rise as the combined result of: (1) an increase in total population, (2) an increase in the proportion of women and of the elderly in the population, since larger amounts of drugs are prescribed for these groups, (3) an increase in the number of patient-physician visits each year, (4) the inclusion of drug coverage in more governmental and private health plans, and (5) an increase in the average price per prescription. Another important factor has been the development of important new drug categories, such as the thiazide diuretics, the oral contraceptives, and both major and minor tranquilizers. Moreover, in almost any version of drug insurance programs enacted, it may be expected that total prescription drug use by the beneficiaries covered would increase from 10 to 15% in the first year, and probably by smaller increments thereafter. It is not known what portion of such an increase under drug insurance would represent meeting previously unmet needs, and what portion would represent program abuse.[9]

While there is much research on NHI and some on drug reimbursement under NHI, there is no data on the impact of NHI on drug R & D. A survey of experts reveals the following as major categories of impact:

1. Depending on deductibles and co-insurance provisions, outpatient service may increase an estimated 30% to 75% while hospital use has been estimated to increase at 5% to 15%.[10] These factors would operate to increase demand for pharmaceuticals and would increase industry profitability. Conversely, reimbursement to nonphysician health care providers and expanded efforts to achieve "rational prescribing" could decrease demand for drugs and reduce industry profitability. Federal payment programs for prescription drugs will also affect market demand for pharmaceuticals. The extent of these effects will depend on federal policy decisions regarding beneficiaries, extent of limitations on covered drugs, patient cost-sharing and reimbursement schemes, and other variables.

[9] Silverman and Lydecker, *op. cit.*, pp. 5–6.

[10] Joseph Newhouse, Charles Phelps, and William Schwartz, *Policy Options and the Impact of National Health Insurance* (Santa Monica, Calif.: Rand Corporation, June, 1974).

2. Increased government, physician, and consumer awareness of health needs resulting from an increase in epidemiological awareness.
3. Greater opportunities for and difficulties in research and clinical trials.

INDUSTRY FORECASTS: THE FUTURE OF THE PHARMACEUTICAL INDUSTRY

One source of information on the future of the pharmaceutical industry is the forecasts of the industry itself. An example of such forecasts is the Pharmaceutical PROSPECTS program of the Futures Group, a futures research firm in Glastonbury, Connecticut, and IMS America, Ltd., a major data-gathering organization in the health field.

The PROSPECTS program uses historical trend data on a number of key aspects of the industry's production, sales, and R & D efforts from which is extrapolated a "surprise-free" projection. This baseline or surprise-free extrapolation assumes that there will be little or no change in upcoming conditions. For example, the baseline extrapolation for R & D expenditures for ethical, human-use drugs suggests an increase from the current level of almost $1,100 million to a 1990 figure of approximately $1,600 million.

Once this extrapolation is established, the program identifies unprecedented events that may alter the extrapolation. These events are identified from published sources, interviews with experts, and PROSPECTS staff members. Each event is then assigned a probability of occurrence for a given year or years to arrive at a cumulative total impact. The probabilities are assigned by the PROSPECTS Advisory Board—a group of leading researchers and decisionmakers in the pharmaceutical industry (see Table 4-4). This process of combining mathematical projections with human judgment about unprecedented future events is called trend impact analysis. The PROSPECTS forecast for pharmaceutical R & D follows.

> Research and development expenditures for ethical, human-use drugs are forecast to continue rising despite reduced productivity of drug research. A number of manufacturers will attempt to reduce research costs as a percentage of sales, but the majority of research-intensive firms are expected to maintain their R & D programs for the next few years. Cost increases from new government regulations and diminished productivity per research dollar may later lead these companies to alter their research-intensive positions.

The cost of research and development for new pharmaceuticals has risen sharply in recent years, and a 7-to-10-year average wait for FDA marketing approval has further reduced the number of companies engaged in basic research. Some large research-oriented pharmaceutical companies have found it difficult to maintain the same level of research as in the past as profit margins and research resources shrink. Product liability costs have led some manufacturers to abandon promising new drugs in research when an adverse reaction (or "abnormal event") is uncovered. One estimate of drug research costs places development of a new drug at $55 million, so the majority of new drug research is undertaken by a relatively small number of laboratories. The number of companies with large research programs has declined and is forecast to drop even further if the present environment continues. The trend away from long-term research projects is especially important: industry is now concentrating increasingly on short-term objectives and existing products. Last year, DuPont devoted 75% of its research budget to existing products, a 12% increase from the previous year. Industry cites the climate of economic uncertainty, the patent law, and government regulation. SmithKline recently analyzed its research program and found negative returns on research during the sales periods 1967 to 1971 and 1972 to 1976.

Since India banned the export of rhesus monkeys in 1978, a shortage of testing animals has increased research costs. This situation will probably be corrected as an American breeding industry emerges and as alternatives to the rhesus are developed. The relevance of animal models for predicting human safety will continue to be controversial and will lead some scientists to search for alternative safety measurements, and to do tests with a variety of species. Computers have been used to evaluate and screen new chemical entities and also to predict the structure of desired compounds. One program recently developed at the University of Mississippi Medical Center describes three-dimension structures of some proteins using amino acid sequences. Researchers are hopeful that the program will lead to the ability to construct medically useful artificial proteins.

Liposomes may have future potential applications in drug delivery systems. Recently, liposomes were used as vehicles to deliver phospholipids to treat respiratory distress syndrome in premature infants. In Europe, researchers have tried to use liposomes for enzyme replacement therapy, but most U.S. investigators are working with cultured cells and laboratory animals. In the future, liposomes may be used to introduce nucleic acids or viruses into cells or even DNA, thus effecting a permanent change in the genetic structure of the recipient cells, although this last application would undoubtedly engender controversy.

Magnetically controlled microspheres are under study as means of delivering concentrated drugs to specific disease sites. Potential applications include treatment of localized cancers and bacterial abscesses. The

Table 4-4. R & D Expenditures for Ethical, Human Use Drugs (Steady Rise Forecast from 1978 Level of Approximately $1.1 Billion to Approximately $1.6 Billion in 1990, in Constant 1975 Dollars)

Event Number	*Forecast*	*Estimated Probability by Year Shown*		*Years to First Impact*	*Years to Maximum Impact*	*Maximum Impact (percent)*
1	Enactment of legislation allowing automatic release of safety and efficacy data after a 5-year exclusive marketing period.	.60	1980	0	5	− 8%
2	Five major pharmaceutical manufacturers abandon basic research and concentrate on drug development: R & D expenditures drop from 10% of sales to 6%.	.20	1985	1	5	−10
3	Trend among U.S. manufacturers to obtain drugs developed by noncompany research (e.g., Upjohn's marketing of Boots's ibuprofen).	.55	1980	1	12	− 4
4	Number of pharmaceutical manufacturers with complete research programs decreases 20% below 1975 levels.	.70	1985	1	5	− 1
5	Establishment of a National Center for Pharmacology (Nelson or Kennedy Bill) to test new drug products for safety, efficacy, and biological availability by government-approved investigators.	.20	1981	2	5	− 2
6	Animal models become available which are better predictors of human efficacy of certain drug products.	.10	1990	1	5	+ 1
7	Animals for drug testing become even more difficult to select: high-cost primates are shown to exhibit symptoms and risks not found in humans.	.65	1980	1	5	+ 1

8	Availability of quantum statistical approach to predict necessary structural features of a compound to produce a specific biological response.	.50	1984	1	10	+ 3
9	Manufacturers are required to establish a plan for postmarketing surveillance of drug experience and utilization for 5 years following the introduction of a new drug.	.80	1980	1	5	+ 1
10	Real costs of developing a single new drug rise 15% over 1975 level (1975 = $12 million average for a new drug).	.70	1985	1	5	+ 2
11	Congressional and public pressure leads to even stricter regulations for INDs and NDAs.	.70	1990	0	5	+ 3
12	R & D costs rise 30% (real growth) leading companies to specialize, narrowing their research activities to a few fields.	.80	1985	1	5	+ 3
13	Availability of computer programs using pattern recognition and cluster analysis to determine the pharmacologic activity of nearly all organic compounds.	.80	1982	1	5	+ 3
14	FDA requires and enforces uniform testing procedures for all nonclinical research (Good Laboratory Practices).	.85	1981	1	5	+ 3
15	FDA requires and enforces good clinical practice standards.	.80	1982	1	5	+ 5
16	Legislation enacted to allow sales of unapproved drugs to a foreign country on its request.	.65	1980	0	3	+ 5
17	Availability of sophisticated drug delivery systems, such as controlled-release implanted, inserted, or surface-applied polymers; magnetically responsive microspheres; use of multiple emulsions; liposomes; etc.	.75	1980	1	5	+ 5

SOURCE: "Research and Development for Ethical, Human Use Drugs," Pharmaceutical PROSPECTS, The Futures Group, and IMS America (August, 1978), p. 13. Used with permission.

method would allow lower doses of drugs to be used and could reduce the adverse effects on other body sites. Sustained release of biochemically active molecules has been demonstrated for more than 100 days with polymer matrices. The technique would probably be used first in bioassays; eventually the polymers may be clinically useful for long-term delivery of macromolecules such as insulin, heparin, and enzymes. The Ocusert disc is one example of a product using controlled release in clinical use today. The disc is a membrane of ethylenevinyl acetate co-polymer about half the size of a contact lens that contains pilocarpine. Thus, the glaucoma drug is delivered directly to the target organ at a controlled rate.

Several pharmaceutical companies have expanded their licensing programs as a means for growth and diversion. A 1972 study showed nearly one-fourth of the top 120 single-entity prescription pharmaceuticals were acquired by their manufacturers from outside sources. Most firms seek products or compounds in exchange for their own agents, although many foreign firms with no U.S. facilities or plans to enter the U.S. market may prefer a licensing agreement with no product exchange. Acquisition is often most practical for gaining research expertise or additional manufacturing capability.

The Drug Regulation Reform Act of 1978 includes a provision allowing U.S. firms to export products not approved by the FDA. Upjohn's injectable contraceptive, Depo-Provera, has frequently been cited as an example of the kind of drug which could be exported if this provision of the bill passes. In that case, a benefit-risk judgment was given as the reason for nonapproval for U.S. marketing. The FDA believed safer alternatives to be widely available in the United States but added that the judgment "is not necessarily appropriate for other countries." If an unapproved drug complies with the requirements of the importing country, the new legislation would permit U.S. manufacturers to export it to that country.[11]

APPENDIX A

NHI Drug Reimbursement Issues and Policy Options

National drug insurance involves a series of complex and interrelated issues that will ultimately affect the drug R & D activity of government

[11] Used with permission from the Futures Group, Pharmaceutical PROSPECTS, and IMS America, "Research and Development for Ethical, Human Use Drugs" (August, 1978), pp. 13–15.

and industry. The issues and corresponding policy options are outlined below.

1. Eligible population
   a. Everyone (universal coverage)
   b. The elderly
   c. Those who are welfare recipients or defined as medically indigent
   d. Those with serious, disabling chronic disease
2. Covered products
   a. All prescription or legend drugs, plus insulin (comprehensive coverage)
   b. All drugs recommended in a voluntary formulary, plus others
   c. Only drugs specified in a compulsory formulary
   d. Mandatory generic dispensing
3. Cost-sharing
   a. No cost-sharing
   b. Fixed co-payment ($1.50 per prescription to be paid by recipient)
   c. Fixed co-insurance (20% of each prescription cost to be paid by recipient)
   d. Annual deductible (including large deductible for catastrophic coverage)
   e. Limitation on number of days supply per prescription
   f. Sliding cost-sharing determined by economic status of patient
4. Acquisition cost reimbursement
   a. Define acquisition cost as average wholesale price (AWP)
   b. Define acquisition cost as actual acquisition cost (AAC)
   c. Define acquisition cost as estimated acquisition cost (EAC)
   d. For multiple-source products, limit reimbursement to maximum allowable cost (MAC) set by program administration
5. Dispensing cost reimbursement
   a. Base dispensing cost on percentage mark-up of acquisition cost
   b. Base dispensing cost on a fixed professional fee
6. Alternative reimbursement approaches
   a. Base reimbursement on "usual and customary" charges
   b. Base reimbursement on annual payment per person (capitation payment)
   c. Base reimbursement on lump sum payments arranged under contract between government and groups of pharmacists

7. Flow of reimbursement funds
   a. Reimbursement in cash to patient
   b. Reimbursement in cash to pharmacist
   c. Government purchase, with replacement of drug supply to pharmacist
8. Data processing
   a. Manual
   b. Electronic
9. Program quality control
   a. No utilization review
   b. Utilization review

APPENDIX B

The Potential Effects of Drug Reimbursement Under NHI on Pharmaceutical R & D

by Michael A. Riddiough

As with most forecasting endeavors, this presentation must be made without good data on which to project trends in pharmaceutical R & D. We make our forecasts about pharmaceutical R & D based on our intuition and a few assumptions. Selected provisions that may be incorporated in NHI will affect the reimbursement and, hence, the use of prescription drugs. I believe the size of various drug markets, which may be affected by NHI, will dictate the future of pharmaceutical R & D. Examples of such provisions include:

- a restricted beneficiary population
- a restricted list of drug benefits (formulary)
- a cost-effective criterion for inclusion in the NHI benefit package
- a cost-sharing responsibility for patients
- a drug wholesale price limitation—at least for multiple source products
- a mechanism to better inform patients about the benefits, risks, and costs of drugs prescribed for their use, e.g., patient package inserts (PPIs)
- postmarketing surveillance
- mandatory use of generic products whenever possible

My assumptions are as follows:

1. In general, a pharmaceutical company's total commitment to R & D is directly related to its total drug sales volume. Therefore, factors that affect drug sales also affect R & D.
2. Pharmaceutical companies specialize in selected areas of therapeutics, and the extent of R & D in a given area of therapeutics is directly proportional to a company's sales in that area. This is not always true but often is (e.g., vaccines).
3. I believe that the factors listed above include the major influences on a company's decisionmaking process that directs its R & D expenditures. I also believe that marketing considerations often outweigh both scientific factors and organizational elements. More specifically, I believe that projected sales and profits from an effort is the overriding factor among all such considerations. Without question, most major companies also are concerned with public welfare, but this is at least a secondary influence to potential profits.

Given these assumptions, the potential effects of various government actions on the size and nature of various drug markets and, in turn, on pharmaceutical R & D are wide-ranging.

Based on very weak evidence, it is estimated that about 1.8 billion outpatient prescriptions and another 1 billion in-hospital prescriptions were filled in 1976. Estimates for total expenditures for prescription drugs range from $12 billion to maybe $15 billion per year. Roughly, on the average, everyone under 65 years of age spends $25 to $60 per year on prescription drugs, and those over 65 spend three times this amount or between $150 to $200 per year.

The vast majority of prescription drugs used in hospitals are paid for by health insurance carriers. Therefore, the person receiving the drug has very little effect on the extent and nature of drug use reimbursement. The in-hospital prescription drug market, approximately 40% of the total market, is directed by physicians, hospital pharmacies, and health insurance carriers, not patients.

Reimbursement for outpatient drug use differs substantially from that of in-hospital use. According to a survey conducted by the National Center for Health Statistics in 1973, about 75% of all outpatient prescription drug acquisitions were paid for totally by the patients taking the drugs. About 13% were purchased completely by insurance carriers, and the remaining 12% by a combination of patients and carriers.

At present, the in-hospital prescription drug market will be affected by any provisions in NHI that affect the purchasing policies of hospital pharmacies and the prescribing habits of physicians, such as drug formularies, not by provisions that may affect patients' willingness to buy drugs such as PPIs.

Because the vast majority of outpatient prescription drug acquisitions are made by patients, the ultimate consumers, this market is more sensitive to factors that affect a person's willingness to take a prescription drug, such as the drug cost and the patient's attitude or knowledge about a given drug.

Since the potential provisions of NIH that may affect prescription drug use and, hence, R & D are widely divergent, it is necessary to consider the possible impact of each separately.

1. No Drug Coverage

No coverage for drugs will probably have little impact on the amount of R & D, although there would probably be some increase in drug sales due to an increase in physician visits and possibly more hospitalization. The direction of R & D, too, will probably show little change, although this depends on the direction of markets created by physicians' prescribing habits and patient demand.

If NIH does not cover drugs, private carriers may do so (barring laws mandating uniform benefits packages in NHI and the private sector). Third-party payers may institute programs to curtail drug use and shape the marketplace with such provisions as formularies.

2. Restricted Beneficiary Population

If the beneficiary population is restricted, the impact on market size will depend on the population selected for coverage. For example, if the elderly are chosen to be covered, then the market is likely to grow because of high drug use among this group and because drug costs will no longer be a limiting factor on drug purchases as is the case now due to the problems of living on fixed incomes. Removal or reduction of drug costs may lead to expanded use of drugs, particularly for chronic conditions.

The market direction also depends on the population chosen. Again, if the elderly are selected, then use of drugs for chronic medical problems such as high blood pressure, arthritis, and central nervous system problems will increase. The direction of R & D will follow the direction of sales.

3. *Restricted Drug Benefits (Formulary)*

Restricted drug benefits could potentially have a very large impact on both the size and the direction of sales and R & D. The use of formularies in NHI would create, direct, and possibly expand markets for selected agents or areas of therapeutics. R & D might then center around these markets. If criteria for inclusion on a NHI formulary includes cost effectiveness, companies may direct their R & D toward those therapeutic markets that need more cost-effective drug therapy and away from those that are saturated with reasonably cost-effective agents.

4. *Patient Cost-sharing Mechanisms*

Cost-sharing mechanisms will have little impact on in-hospital drug use because patients seldom pay for such use. Therefore, cost-sharing will have little impact on R & D. The effect of cost-sharing on outpatient drug use depends on the level of co-payment. If co-payments are high and are meaningful to the patient, then demand for drugs may be limited more to those agents deemed necessary by the patient. Low co-payments will probably not affect drug use very much, and patient demand, not necessarily need, will dictate the size and direction of the market. By themselves, patient cost-sharing mechanisms will probably have minimal effect on pharmaceutical R & D.

5. *Wholesale Price Limitation: Maximum Allowable Cost (MAC) Program*

The impact of a MAC program depends on the mix of single-source brand name products and multiple-source generic products sold by a company. In general, companies with large R & D budgets are the major producers of single-source brand name products. Some of these companies also produce generic or "branded generic" products and compete with producers of other generic products for given therapeutic markets. Programs like MAC attempt to limit the wholesale price of multiple-source products purchased by government programs, including Medicare and Medicaid. MAC may not affect the total revenue of those companies producing both single-source and multiple-source products because whatever revenue that may be lost as a result of restricted prices on multiple-source products sold to the government is likely to be recouped through increased prices of single-source and multiple-source products sold in the private sector.

The effect of MAC and similar programs on R & D may depend on how a company allocates profits from sales of multiple-source products. Most multiple-source products are off-patent, and little R & D is devoted to them unless a company is creating a new market for such products. If a company's R & D program depends on sales from its multiple-source drugs, then theoretically programs like MAC could hinder its R & D incentives. If a company funds its R & D through sales of single-source products, as I believe to be the more common situation, then MAC will probably not stymie its R & D program. MAC could, however, discourage manufacturers of primarily multiple-source products from mounting large R & D programs.

6. Improved Patient Education

Possibly the biggest threat to the current *modus operandi* of the pharmaceutical industry is a growing uneasiness about prescription drugs among the consumer population. I believe many people are asking more questions about the drugs they are asked to take. I think their concerns are based on possible adverse effects and sometimes on cost. Quite simply, people want to know what a drug will do for them—or to them. Congress is contemplating legislation that will expand the use of PPIs in order to help people better understand the drugs they are taking. No one knows what effect PPIs will have on either patients' knowledge about drugs or their use of them.

The remaining item, postmarketing surveillance, needs attention, but at this point its impact is less clear than the impact of the other six items.

All of the possibilities mentioned above either have been or will be included in discussions of drug coverage under NHI. All of them are interactive; that is, each can affect one or more of the others. For example, a cost-effectiveness criterion for inclusion of a drug on a formulary combined with an effective mechanism to educate consumers of prescription drugs about benefits, costs, and risks could be a powerful incentive for manufacturers to enhance their products' safety and efficacy.

No one knows for sure what impact drug coverage under NHI will have on pharmaceutical R & D. If controls are loose and the market expands and all other factors remain constant, then R & D should at least stay the same if not increase. NHI provisions affecting the markets for products in selected areas of therapeutics will influence the extent and direction of R & D in each of those areas.

HIGHLIGHTS OF THE DISCUSSION

The discussion at the Foresight Seminar on the Impact of National Health Insurance (NHI) on Pharmaceutical R & D was led by Peter Goldschmidt of Policy Research Inc., Michael A. Riddiough of the Health Program of the Office of Technology Assessment, and John Virts, a corporate economist with Eli Lilly & Company.

The discussion pointed out the difficulty and importance of considering the links between NHI, drug R & D, and health outcomes. While there was general agreement that drug sales will increase with NHI, even with MAC limitations, no clear link was drawn between MAC and increased R & D expenditures or breakthroughs in specific categories.

In considering the future of drug R & D, the group used a variety of charts developed by the Pharmaceutical PROSPECTS program to review the range of events that might encourage or discourage R & D expenditures in the United States (see Table 4-4). Each chart provided events, estimates of the likelihood that the events will occur by a certain year, the number of years until their first impact is felt, the years to maximum impact, and the potential maximum impact on the aggregate level of R & D spending for each event.

In examining a forecast that R & D expenditures would rise from $1.1 billion to $1.6 billion by 1990 (in constant dollars), the group agreed that corporate finance, public and political pressures, inflation-driven increases in R & D costs, and breakthroughs in the methods of drug delivery would be as or even more important than national health insurance in shaping drug R & D expenditures.

The group agreed that NHI in some form is likely but that its impact will be contingent on several of the specific provisions listed in Appendix A of this chapter. These provisions include method of reimbursement (whether for everyone or for specific categories of people such as children or the elderly), the existence of price controls such as MAC, and the degree of co-payment.

Participants were particularly interested in three questions related to NHI and drug R & D: (1) appropriate utilization of drug therapies, (2) ways in which cost containment would affect new drugs, and (3) incentives for significant innovation in drug R & D.

Disagreement arose over the effect of reviews of drug utilization that might accompany NHI. Some felt that it would provide positive feedback and cause doctors to use their judgment more effectively; others felt such reviews would stifle doctors' judgments.

Participants noted that NHI is primarily a financing mechanism rather than a conscious approach to improving health therapies and that its influence on drug R & D might not be directly translatable into the discovery of new or better drugs. Some argued that health maintenance organizations (HMOs) would have a more important impact than NHI on development of effective therapies. Others argued that NHI—particularly with utilization reviews—would provide greater insights into therapeutic effectiveness and ultimately hasten drug R & D breakthroughs. Participants familiar with the drug industry claimed that much current innovative research is funded by the profits from drugs that would be covered by MAC limitations, and, therefore, MAC limitations would result in a decrease in R & D expenditures. Others countered that this might force effort away from me-too drugs toward those with high therapeutic gain.

In order to evaluate the significance of drug R & D on health outcomes and health expenditures, the group considered the impact that a moratorium on new drugs would have and where the most important breakthroughs were likely to take place. One indicator—the average age at death—would not be affected significantly since there is only a small proportion of cases where life could be extended by drugs. Yet the group thought that in the next few years new drugs would have a small but important effect on morbidity—days of impaired functioning—and that the magnitude of this effect would increase as the population ages.

Participants felt that the areas of the greatest need and the greatest likelihood of drug breakthroughs were, first, the cardiovascular area and, second, the category that includes neoplasms, the endocrine system, and metabolic diseases. Yet the group felt that a paradoxical result would emerge: drug breakthroughs in the neoplasm/endocrine/metabolic and the cardiovascular areas, in that order, would lead both to the greatest savings and the greatest increases in health care costs. Drug breakthroughs, the discussion suggested, would reduce health care costs when they prevented illness or replaced more costly therapies presently in use. Conversely, they would increase health care costs when they provided therapies where none existed before and when they prolonged lives, particularly among the elderly. Thus, some of these breakthroughs would keep those most in need of medical care alive longer, increasing costs as well as health.

5
The National Center for Drug Science: Policy Questions and Long-term Consequences

The Drug Regulation Reform Act of 1979 contains a provision that would establish a National Center for Drug Science to encourage greater training for health providers in the proper use of drugs, to provide an annual assessment of drug use in the United States, and to develop policy and scientific research on drugs, including development of "orphan" drugs. This chapter will explore the proposed major functions of the center, the need for establishing a new center to perform them, and the potential long-term consequences of doing so.

THE DRUG REGULATION REFORM ACT OF 1979

The Drug Regulation Reform Act of 1979, S.1075 and H.R. 11611, 96th Congress, represented the culmination of several years of effort on the part of members of Congress, the administration, industry, academic researchers, and consumer activists. It called for a major revision of the way in which new drugs are brought onto the market and included provisions for surveillance of these drugs after marketing. These and a variety of other issues are dealt with in Title I of the Act, a digest of which appears in Appendix A, page 97. Many of the proposed changes, particularly postmarketing surveillance, are related to the operation of the center proposed in Title II.

The advancement of science and public policy related to drug research and drug regulation has been an ongoing concern within the academic community, industry, and government. Several government task forces, advisory boards, and private working conferences have endorsed the concept of scientific and policy research in the health care system. These groups have supported one or more approaches to a drug science board that would develop methodology for integrating premarketing and postmarketing requirements for regulation, propose standards of bioequivalence or bioavailability, and deal with numerous other research questions. Proponents of simultaneous research on drug science and drug policy argue that neither the FDA nor the NIH has addressed these issues adequately.

Title II of S. 1075 would establish a National Center for Drug Science. In earlier versions of the bill, the center was called the National Center for Clinical Pharmacology. The most recent version, passed by the Senate in September, 1979, may undergo further changes (see Appendix B, page 98).

The center is intended to be a focal point for thinking and research on the drug therapy system. It would provide the intelligence and guidance for scientific and policy research on the use of drugs. It would also conduct and support research on safety and efficacy, facilitate research breakthroughs, and test for "orphan" drugs—drugs for diseases whose incidence is too small to make the drug commercially viable. It would also develop a program to analyze drug innovation, assessment, and utilization and to monitor and evaluate the impact of regulation. The center would issue periodic reports on disease areas requiring further research commitments as well as on promising lines of research. It would prepare an annual drug experience assessment report with recommendations for improved drug use. Finally, the center would support training and continuing education in clinical pharmacology and clinical pharmacy for physicians, pharmacists, and other health care providers.

A primary question, however, is whether a new federal center is really needed.

Scientific Research on Drugs

Scientific research focuses on what a scientist must know to discover new drugs or explore their effects within the body and on what a practitioner must know to use drug therapies effectively. For the purposes of this discussion, research on drugs involves clinical and laboratory investigation of scientific breakthroughs and of pharmacologic and therapeutic effects of drugs and actual testing of drugs and drug products.

Beyond the commitment to resolve thorny scientific questions, additional avenues of investigation at the center would include facilitating breakthroughs in important basic or applied research into drug therapies and testing of specific new drugs needed for diseases or conditions of low incidence. Breakthrough support is needed to ensure that important new leads are pursued, since both industry and academia are sometimes unable to do this. The rationale for "orphan" drug testing lies in the fact that, although such testing is conducted on a minor scale by the NIH, universities, and some companies, these efforts do not represent a substantial commitment to those diseases of low incidence for which drug therapies may hold promise.

Policy Research on Drugs

Policy research, often based on scientific research, deals with what a government decisionmaker must know in order to allocate resources or establish regulatory procedures. Drug-related policy research seeks to inform decisionmakers about how to target research funds. Policy research at the center would also include gathering information on the impact of regulation on drug innovation, finding methods of improving the processes of drug research, development, approval, and utilization, and establishing risk/benefit calculations for determining safety and efficacy. The FDA conducts some policy research, but it cannot promote policy research on drug discovery. The NIH does not have major responsibility for performing this function. Therefore, it is proposed that responsibility for policy research be formerly vested in the center.

Training in Clinical Pharmacology and Clinical Pharmacy

The center would work to strengthen and supplement the training of physicians and other health professionals in the use of drug therapies. Specifically, the center would support the development of training programs in schools of medicine, osteopathy, dentistry, pharmacy, podiatry, nursing, and allied health professions. Such programs would include clinical pharmacology and clinical pharmacy courses for full-time students as well as continuing education, traineeships, and fellowships.

Most observers support the need for such training, though some have questioned whether HEW units already involved in medical education could not handle this function.

COSTS AND AREAS OF IMPACT OF THE CENTER

S.1075 authorizes funds for scientific research, policy research, and drug experience assessment that rise from $5 million the first year of operation to $9 million the third year. Funds for training functions range from about $13 million the first year to about $15 million the third year. If these figures were extrapolated for the sake of discussion, during the first 10 years the research and assessment work of the center would cost $100 to $120 million, and the training functions would cost $180 to $200 million.

While the relationship between the center's work and the areas listed below is not clear, the center could have an impact, either positive or negative, on them. The amounts give some indication of the magnitude of expenditures. The inconsistencies and controversies surrounding the figures and the absence of figures for some areas point out the need for policy research.

- overall health R & D in the United States—$5.526 billion in 1977[1]
- federal health R & D expenditures—$3.351 billion in 1977[2]
- drug R & D expenditures by the NIH for the period from 1959 to 1974—estimates of expenditures of the 11 units of the NIH for drug R & D ranged from $650 million to $1 billion[3]
- health R & D expenditures by the NIH—$2.244 billion in 1977[4]
- industry expenditures for drug R & D—$1.5 billion for 1978[5]
- cost of discovery and development of a new drug—estimates vary widely; although $30 to $40 million is a plausible range, recent studies suggest $54 million (see Chapter 3)
- number and cost of drugs prescribed—1.4 billion prescriptions were dispensed by community pharmacies in 1978 and approximately 1.2 billion by hospital pharmacies in 1974; retail sales of prescriptions in community pharmacies were estimated at $7 to $8 billion in 1977 (see Chapter 4)

[1]*NIH Factbook* (Washington, D.C.: Government Printing Office, 1978), p. 4.

[2]*Ibid.*, p. 4.

[3]Edward J. Burger, "The Current Role of the Federal Government in Drug Related R & D: What Is It and What Should It Be?" *Impact of Public Policy on Drug Innovation and Pricing*, eds. Samuel A. Mitchell and Emery A. Link (Washington, D.C.: The American University, 1976), p. 395.

[4]*NIH Factbook, op. cit.*, p. 4.

[5]Pharmaceutical Manufacturers Association, *Annual Report, 1978* (Washington, D.C.: PMA, 1978).

- drugs prescribed unnecessarily and cost of adverse drug reactions—(no adequate data at a national level)
- potential growth in consumer expenditures for drugs—drug expenditures are likely to rise from current levels to between $13.4 and $24 billion in the year 2000 depending on assumptions;[6] per capita national health expenditures for drugs and drug sundries are forecast to rise from $57 in 1977 to between $80 and $95 in 1990 depending on drug prices, insurance coverage, generic dispensing, and other factors[7]

POTENTIAL LONG-TERM CONSEQUENCES OF THE NATIONAL CENTER FOR DRUG SCIENCE

The following is a preliminary list of major categories that may be affected by establishment of the center and in what areas the effects may be felt.

Consumers

- increased awareness of risks and benefits of drug therapies
- greater reservoir of knowledge for consumer group action
- diminished level of adverse drug reactions

Physicians

- greater awareness of the risks and benefits of drug therapies
- altered prescribing behavior
- increased knowledge of drug interactions

Industry

- marketing strategies
- expenditures for research (discovering new drugs)
- expenditures for development (seeking FDA marketing approval)
- types of new drugs sought
- number of new drugs discovered
- number and type of new drugs developed for marketing
- anticipatory drug assessment

[6]Selma J. Mushkin *et al.*, "Cost of Disease and Illness in the United States in the Year 2000," *Public Health Reports*, Vol. 93, No. 5 (September-October, 1978), pp. 493–588.

[7]The Futures Group, Pharmaceutical PROSPECTS, and IMS America, "Research and Development for Ethical, Human Use Drugs" (August, 1978), pp. 11–12.

- research and marketing benefits from drug experience assessment report

Federal government

FDA:

- could allow new drugs easier market entry because of postmarketing surveillance and assessment
- could make market entry of new drugs more difficult because of standard of comparative efficacy that emerges from the center's assessment of drugs in use
- could force companies to test for unapproved use where the drug experience assessment report shows such uses
- additional testing or labeling requirements may result from the center's work

NIH:

- altered research priorities

HEW:

- medicaid and other reimbursement for most risk-free drugs

Academic research community

- interdisciplinary efforts in scientific and policy research on drugs
- greater understanding of systemic effects of classes of drugs

Availability of prescription drugs

- sales in particular drug categories
- prescribing (and sales) of drugs in particular categories
- categories likely to be most affected: antibiotics, psychotropic drugs, and hormones
- number of therapeutically significant new drugs marketed

Pharmaceutical R & D in general

- drug production approaches, e.g., genetic alteration
- drug delivery mechanism breakthroughs, e.g., controlled-release polymers, magnetically responsive microspheres, and liposomes

APPENDIX A

Digest of Title I of the Drug Regulation Reform Act of 1979, S.1075

Prohibits the manufacture, importation, export, or distribution of a drug entity or a drug product without the prior issuance by the Department of Health, Education, and Welfare of a monograph containing a description of such drug and requirements and guidelines for the contents of information labeling for the forms of drug products eligible for licensing under such monograph.

Authorizes the Secretary of Health, Education, and Welfare to require, in a monograph, postmarketing surveillance of any drug, old or new, for a period of up to five years. Limits the issuance of such monographs to drugs determined safe and effective. Defines "safe" as meaning the health benefits of the drug entity or product clearly outweigh the risks it presents, taking into account pertinent standards and requirements. Defines "effective" to mean that a drug entity when incorporated into a drug product used in accordance with the use conditions set forth on the drug label, will have the effect represented. Provides for amendment, suspension, or revocation of a monograph under specified conditions.

Authorizes the provisional issuance of a monograph (for a period not to exceed five years) for any drug entity intended to be used in treatment of a life-threatening or severely debilitating disease when: (1) no other effective methods of treatment exist; or, (2) such drug entity offers a major advantage to patients compared to the benefits of alternative methods; and, (3) delaying issuance would present significantly greater risks to patients affected by such disease. Requires significant evidence of effectiveness and safety for such provisional issuance.

Establishes a monograph-petition review procedure requiring a public hearing on the issuance, amendment, or revocation of any monograph, followed by a review of the evidence and issued by a drug science advisory committee, whose recommendations shall be forwarded to the Secretary for his final decision. Authorizes judicial review of a final order of the Secretary by a United States Court of Appeal.

Requires, with specified exceptions, the registration of domestic and foreign establishments engaged in the manufacture, import, export, or distribution of any drug entity or drug product.

Prohibits for five years after the issuance date of a monograph the licensure of any drug product without: (1) written authorization from the monograph petitioner; or, (2) data and information independent of the monograph which would support a determination that the monograph could be issued. Permits the licensure of a drug product, after the expiration of such five-year period, without the making of necessary animal and clinical studies already made to demonstrate the safety and efficacy of the drug product under the original monograph.

Requires registration of any drug to be used in a drug investigation, and revocation of registration if the human participants in the investigation are subject to unreasonable and significant risk of illness or injury. Specifies standards and requirements for such investigations. Requires the informed consent of participants in such investigations unless the immediate use of the drug product is, in the investigator's opinion, needed to preserve the participant's life and time is not sufficient to obtain either consent from either the participant or his legal representative.

Authorizes the Secretary to: (1) issue written guidelines regarding protocols and methods for conducting investigations; and, (2) review and advise, upon request, regarding specified aspects of a drug investigation.

Requires unlicensed drug products and drug entities not subject to monographs to obtain permits for export to foreign countries. Specifies requirements for such exports.

Exempts homeopathic drug entities and products from monograph, licensure, and investigational use requirements if manufactured or imported in accordance with import/export registration requirements of this Act.

Requires: (1) patient information labeling in laypersons' language of the risks, benefits, side effects, and so forth of any drug entity or product; and, (2) practitioner information labeling that identifies the licensee, registrant, permittee, and manufacturer of such drug.

APPENDIX B

Title II of the Drug Regulation Reform Act of 1979, S.1075

TITLE II—NATIONAL CENTER FOR DRUG SCIENCE

Amendment to Public Health Service Act

Sec. 201. The Public Health Service Act is amended by inserting after title XVII the following new title:

TITLE XVIII—NATIONAL CENTER FOR DRUG SCIENCE

Establishment of Center

Sec. 1801. (a) There is established in the Department of Health, Education, and Welfare an office which shall be known as the National Center for Drug Science (hereinafter in this title referred to as the "Center"). The Center shall have a Division of Policy and Research, which shall be responsible for carrying out the functions described in section 1802, and a Division of Clinical Pharmacology and Clinical Pharmacy Training, which shall be responsible for carrying out the functions described in sections 1803 and 1804. The Center shall be under the direction of the Director of the Center (hereinafter in this title referred to as the "Director") who shall be appointed by the Secretary. The Director shall be classified at grade GS-18 of the General Schedule.

(b) To implement this title, the Director may, in addition to any other authority available to him, use personnel, equipment, and facilities and other physical resources of the Department of Health, Education, and Welfare. The Director may secure for the Center, for such periods as the Director deems advisable, the assistance and advice of experts and consultants from the United States and abroad in accordance with section 3109, title 5, United States Code, and to compensate individuals so employed for each day (including traveltime) at rates not in excess of the maximum rate of pay for grade GS-18 as provided in section 5332 of title 5, United States Code, and, while such experts and consultants are so serving away from their homes or regular places of business, to pay such employees travel expenses and per diem in lieu of subsistence at rates authorized by section 5703 of title 5, United States Code, for persons in Government service employed intermittently. The Director may hold conferences and meetings, and undertake other activities consistent with the functions of the Center, when appropriate.

Policy and Research Functions of the Center

Sec. 1802. (a)(1) In accordance with the procedures set forth in paragraph (2), the Center may, upon request or on its initiative, conduct and support research, including investigations—

(A) of the safety and effectiveness of drugs approved by the Food and Drug Administration;

(B) for the development of drugs for diseases and other conditions of low incidence; and

(C) to facilities breakthroughs in drug science research.

(2) Prior to conducting or supporting research under subparagraph (B) or (C) of paragraph (1), the Center shall—

(A) publish, in the Federal Register, a notice which shall contain a statement that the Center intends to conduct or support such research and such notice shall include the objectives of such research, the nature of the drug, if any, which would be the subject of such research, and those findings required to be made under subparagraph (B),

(B) find that—

(i) the research is of special significance;

and

(ii) there is either no or minimal research of a similar nature currently being conducted outside of government or by other agencies of government, either directly or by grant or contract.

(3) The director shall periodically report to the Secretary on (1) promising areas of any new techniques in drug science research and (2) diseases or other conditions for which current research on drugs is insufficient.

(b) The Center shall conduct an ongoing program of drug science policy research, either directly or by grant or contract. The Center, in conducting such a research, shall review, analyze, and where appropriate make recommendations and reports to the Secretary regarding the relationship of drugs to the public health, including:

(1) the impact of regulation on drug innovation and development;

(2) problems inherent in the analysis of risks and benefits, the formulation of risk versus benefit ratios, and the use of such ratios in approving drugs; and

(3) methods for improving and accelerating the overall drug research, innovation, development, investigation, approval, and utilization process.

(c) The Center shall conduct an ongoing review and analysis of the use of drugs in the United States (as determined on the basis of information submitted under the Federal Food, Drug, and Cosmetic Act and other information obtained by the Secretary) and on the basis of such review and analysis prepare an annual Drug Experience Assessment Report for the Secretary. The report may be on such categories of drugs as the Director determines is appropriate. The report shall include, for the drugs included in the report, a qualitative analysis of the use of such drugs as are currently in use in the United States, adverse effects and unanticipated reactions from such drugs, an assessment of the frequency of the occurrence of such effects and reactions, an analysis of the use of such drugs on a regional basis, by specialties of medicine, or any other category of use of such drugs and shall include recommendations for improvement in the use of such drugs.

(d) The Director shall publish and otherwise make available to the public the reports submitted under this section.

(e) There are authorized to be appropriated to carry out the purposes of this section $5,000,000 for the fiscal year ending September 30, 1981,

$7,000,000 for the fiscal year ending September 30, 1982, and $9,000,000 for the fiscal year ending September 30, 1983.

Training Functions of the Center: Grants for Programs in Clinical Pharmacology and Clinical Pharmacy

Sec. 1803. (a)(1) From funds appropriated under paragraph (2) the Director may make grants—

(A) to schools of medicine, osteopathy, dentistry, pharmacy, podiatry, and nursing and to groups of such schools for—

(i) the planning, establishment, and operation of new programs; and

(ii) the expansion of existing programs of training in clinical pharmacology for full-time students (as defined in section 770(c)(2) or 810(d)(2)) enrolled in such schools;

(B) to training centers for allied health professions for—

(i) the planning, establishment, and operation of new programs; and

(ii) the expansion of existing programs of training in clinical pharmacology for students enrolled in such centers; and

(C) to schools of pharmacy for—

(i) the planning, establishment, and operation of new programs; and

(ii) the expansion of existing programs of training in clinical pharmacy for full-time students (as defined in section 770(c)(2)) enrolled in such schools.

(2) There are authorized to be appropriated for payments under grants under this subsection $3,000,000 for the fiscal year ending September 30, 1981, $4,000,000 for the fiscal year ending September 30, 1982, and $5,000,000 for the fiscal year ending September 30, 1983.

(b)(1) From funds appropriated under paragraph (2), the Director may make grants to schools of medicine, osteopathy, dentistry, pharmacy, podiatry, and nursing and to other public and nonprofit private entities for the planning, establishment, and operation of new programs, and for the expansion of existing programs, of continuing education in clinical pharmacology and clinical pharmacy for physicians, dentists, pharmacists, podiatrists, and nurses.

(2) There are authorized to be appropriated for payments under grants under this subsection $2,000,000 for the fiscal year ending September 30, 1981, $3,000,000 for the fiscal year ending September 30, 1982, and $4,000,000 for the fiscal year ending September 30, 1983.

(c)(1) From funds appropriated under paragraph (2), the Director may make grants to or enter into contracts with public and nonprofit private entities for demonstration projects to demonstrate new roles for (A) clinical pharmacologists and clinical pharmacists in the practice of medicine, osteopathy, dentistry, pharmacy, podiatry, and nursing and (B) clinical pharmacology in nursing.

(2) There are authorized to be appropriated for payments under grants or contracts under this subparagraph $1,000,000 for the fiscal year ending September 30, 1981, $1,500,000 for the fiscal year ending September 30, 1982, and $2,000,000 for the fiscal year ending September 30, 1983.

(d)(1) No grant may be made or contract entered into under this section unless an application therefor has been submitted to, and approved by, the Director. Such application shall be in such form, submitted in such manner, and contain such information, as the Director shall by regulation prescribe. The Director may approve or disapprove any application for a grant or contract under this title but only after consultation with the National Advisory Council on Drug Science established by section 1805.

(2) The amount of any grant or contract under this section shall be determined by the Director. Contracts may be entered into under this section without regard to sections 3648 and 3709 of the Revised Statutes (31 U.S.C. 529; 41 U.S.C. 5). Payments of any such grant or contract may be made in advance or by way of reimbursement and in such installments and on such conditions as the Director deems necessary to carry out the purposes of this section.

Traineeships and Fellowships

Sec. 1804. (a)(1) From funds appropriated under subsection (b)(1) the Director may make grants to schools of medicine, osteopathy, dentistry, pharmacy, podiatry, and nursing for the provision of traineeships to assist physicians, dentists, pharmacists, podiatrists, nurses, and other qualified individuals in meeting the cost of obtaining graduate training and research training in clinical pharmacology and clinical pharmacy.

(2) From funds appropriated under subsection (b)(2), the Director may provide fellowships to physicians, dentists, pharmacists, podiatrists, nurses, and other qualified individuals to undertake research at the Center. The Secretary shall provide sabbatical leave in accordance with section 5701(c), title 5, United States Code, and otherwise assist scientists and other qualified individuals (notwithstanding whether such person is classified within the senior executive service) employed by the Department of Health, Education, and Welfare in obtaining such fellowships.

(3) No grant for traineeships and fellowships may be made under this section unless an application therefor has been submitted to, and approved by, the Director. Such application shall be in such form, be submitted in such manner, and contain such information, as the Director may prescribe. Traineeships and fellowships under such a grant shall be awarded in accordance with such regulations as the Secretary shall pre-

scribe. The amount of any such grant shall be determined by the Director.

(b)(1) There are authorized to be appropriated for payments under grants under paragraph (1) of subsection (1) $2,000,000 for the fiscal year ending September 30, 1981, $2,500,000 for the fiscal year ending September 30, 1982, and $3,000,000 for the fiscal year ending September 30, 1983.

(2) There are authorized to be appropriated for fellowships under paragraph (2) of subsection (a) $500,000 for the fiscal year ending September 30, 1981, $600,000 for the fiscal year ending September 30, 1982, and $700,000 for the fiscal year ending September 30, 1983.

(c) Traineeships and fellowships provided under this subsection shall include such stipends and allowances (including travel and subsistence expenses and dependency allowances) as the Director may deem necessary.

National Advisory Board

Sec. 1805. (a)(1) There is established a board to be known as the National Advisory Board on Drug Science (hereinafter in this section referred to as the "Board"). The Board shall consult with, advise, and make recommendations to the Director with respect to the responsibilities prescribed by this title, and shall review and comment upon the activities of the Center.

(2) The Board shall be composed of fifteen members appointed by the Secretary, four of whom shall be appointed from the general public to represent the consumers of health care. In determining who shall be a member of the Board, the Secretary shall solicit recommendations from the National Academy of Science.

(b)(1) Members of the Board shall be appointed for a term of three years, except that any member appointed to fill a vacancy occurring prior to the expiration of the term for which the member's predecessor was appointed shall be appointed for the remainder of such term. No member shall be removed, except for cause. Members may be reappointed to the Board.

(2) Members of the Board (other than members who are officers or employees of the United States), while attending meetings or conferences thereof or otherwise serving on the business of the Board, shall be entitled to receive for each day (including traveltime) in which they are so serving the daily equivalent of the annual rate of basic pay in effect for grade GS-18 of the General Schedule; and while so serving away from their homes or regular places of business. All members may be allowed travel expenses, including per diem in lieu of subsistence, as authorized by section 5703(b) of title 5, United States Code, for persons in the Government service employed intermittently.

(c) Section 14 of the Federal Advisory Committee Act shall not apply with respect to the Board.

HIGHLIGHTS OF THE DISCUSSION

Participants at the session identified policy questions surrounding the establishment of the National Center for Drug Science (see Figure 5-1) and focused on some of its potential impacts (see Figure 5-2). The overall position of the speakers—John Burns, vice president for research of Hoffmann-La Roche, Marcia Greenberger, director of the Women's Rights Project of the Center for Law and Social Policy, and John Oates, professor of medicine and pharmacology at Vanderbilt University School of Medicine—was generally favorable toward the center, with some reservations.

Participants discussed the advantages, risks, and possible alternatives to the proposed center.

The advantages of the proposed center that were identified included the following:

1. Professionalism

The center would provide for a high level of scientific professionalism across many disciplines concerned with drug research and use. The center would facilitate communication and planning among academic, government, corporate, and consumer groups and would do so at very little financial cost.

A current problem in drug research is the lack of adequate professional support due to low or nonexistent government loans and stipends for research education. The center would encourage better recruitment and career support for researchers just entering the field. Moreover, establishment of the center would symbolize the government's commitment to drug problems and help attract better scientists to this area of specialization.

Finally, the center would encourage greater communication across national boundaries by serving as a communication and information link with international drug groups, researchers, and suppliers. More information would be available about drugs not currently researched or used in the United States.

2. Research

The center would provide for a broad look at drug use, drug efficacy, side effects, and public health problems in relation to drug R & D. Such long-range and broad research and planning are not currently

Section 1801 Establishment of the Center

Relationship to*
  industry
  university researchers
  other governmental units
To be part of NIH, FDA, or separate

Section 1802 Scientific Research, Policy Research, and Drug Experience Assessment Report

Research on Safety and Efficacy*
  standards of comparative effectiveness
Orphan Drug Research
  prevalence and forecasts for diseases of low incidence
  marketing of drugs discovered; patent protection
Facilitating Breakthroughs*
  how best accomplished
  confidentiality of grant applications, scientific information, trade secrets
Federal Register Notice of Center's Intent to Research a Disease Area
  Center able to verify or dispute others' claims
Periodic Publication of the Center's Work
  most appropriate ways to gather and release information
Policy Research
  how these reports will be made public
The Drug Experience Assessment Report
  comprehensiveness of drug categories covered over time
  cost of the assessment
Making Public the Results of the Center's Work
  effectiveness for consumers and consumer groups
Authorizing Funding Levels
  is $9 million a year adequate?
  staffing and equipping the center

Section 1803 Training Functions of the Center

How Best Accomplished

Figure 5-1. Policy questions on the functioning of the National Center for Drug Science. (Asterisks indicate areas of greatest interest to seminar participants.)

incorporated into any existing programs. The center would permit long-term research projects that are now limited by short-term grants. Research might focus on such areas as the search for drugs that are more effective with fewer and less dangerous side effects, toxicology of specific drugs, applicability of particular drug findings from animal subjects to humans, and availability of particular drugs worldwide.

3. Consumer Protection

The proposed center would serve as a clearinghouse for information on drug use, abuse, and benefits to the public. Studies show that public awareness does lead to better use of drugs. If the people are

1. On Consumers
   awareness of risks and benefits of drug therapies*
   greater reservoir of knowledge for consumer group action
   diminished level of adverse drug reactions
   overuse of drugs*

2. On Physicians
   greater awareness of the risks and benefits of drug therapies*
   altered prescribing behavior*
   increased knowledge of drug interactions*

3. On Industry
   marketing strategies
   expenditures for research (discovering new drugs)*
   expenditures for development (seeking FDA marketing approval)*
   types of new drugs sought*
   number of new drugs discovered*
   number and types of new drugs developed for marketing
   anticipatory drug assessment
   research and marketing benefits from drug experience assessment report
   duplication of clinical research*

4. On the Federal Government

   (FDA)
   easier market entry because of postmarketing surveillance and assessment*
   harder market entry because of standard of comparative efficacy*
   burden of testing by companies for unapproved use shown by the drug experience assessment report*
   other testing or labeling requirements resulting from the center's work

   (NIH)
   altered research priorities*

   (HEW)
   Medicaid and other reimbursement for most risk-free drugs*
   relative productivity of government and industry research*

5. On Academic Research Community
   interdisciplinary efforts in scientific and policy research on drugs*
   greater understanding of systemic effects of classes of drugs*

6. On Prescription Drugs
   on sales in particular drug categories
   on prescribing (and sales) of drugs in particular categories*
   categories to be most affected, e.g., antibiotics
   number of therapeutically significant new drugs marketed*

7. On Pharmaceutical R & D in General
   drug production approaches, e.g., genetic alteration
   drug delivery mechanism breakthroughs, e.g., controlled-release polymers
   orphan drugs*
   third-world drug needs*

Figure 5-2. Potential impacts of the National Center for Drug Science. (Asterisks indicate areas of greatest interest to seminar participants.)

aware of the risks of certain drugs, they can make more careful decisions about drug use. Through advertising, in-house publications, and other public education channels, the center would prepare the public for more effective drug use.

A further protection for the public is the improved education of physicians. As physicians are provided with better information about the availability, risks, and benefits of the drugs they prescribe, they are in a better position to prescribe those drugs wisely.

The concerns or disadvantages of the center as discussed by participants included the following:

1. Replication

A large number of participants expressed concern that the proposed center would replicate programs already in existence and that if new funding were not clearly specified for the center its establishment could lead to the loss of funding now committed to valuable research programs. Some argued that mechanisms for achieving the center's objectives already exist; what is needed is designated responsibility and a heightened priority within existing institutions rather than the creation of a new administrative structure. Participants suggested that the proposed center be designed to supplement, rather than replace, existing programs.

2. Deregulation

Public opinion generally favors less, rather than more, regulation. This attitude is somewhat modified in regard to drugs, because the public wants higher safety standards for drugs. Bureaucratic bias toward safety versus benefits results in long delays in marketing a drug and the center might make the delays worse. Some participants questioned whether a certain degree of risk might be warranted for drugs that have proven or potential benefits; that is, people should have the option of taking risks if they wish to secure the benefits of new drugs. One proposed solution to this dilemma was to ensure that the postmarket surveillance include an analysis of whether delays to ensure safety were worth the costs.

3. Centralization

There was some concern that the centralized structure of the proposed center would endanger the dissemination of information to a variety of groups across the United States.

To achieve balance in the location of its functions, some participants felt that the central coordinating role should be in Washington, D.C.; but in order to contribute effectively to research and training in the drug sciences and to have an impact on physician education, the drug science center must allocate substantial support to extramural programs which have a direct influence on the education and recruitment process and which bring a diversity of innovation to the field. It was suggested that it might be better to have a larger, more widespread structure, such as a network of hospitals and laboratories, to carry on the center's activities in order to spread the activities and findings across a wider range of people.

Similarly, concern was expressed that the center could become too centralized in specialty areas; it could separate disciplines by pigeonholeing them into administrative units. One proposed solution was to have an advisory council or board to oversee the activities of the center's diverse units and to encourage cooperative efforts and planning.

Finally, the center might cause considerable confusion by combining the functions of existing agencies into one central structure. The participants felt that a clear distinction should be drawn among existing programs and the proposed center or, alternatively, the new center should be incorporated into one of the existing programs.

4. Naïveté

Concern was expressed that the center's objectives have been tried a number of times before to no avail. Perhaps the problem is inherent in drug use, which includes inevitable hazards. No structure can prevent such risks and still permit drug use.

Furthermore, in regard to consumer information about drugs, many patients are not qualified to evaluate a particular drug. Providing partial information to the patients who lack a physician's knowledge could cause patients to discontinue use of drugs to their own detriment. Physicians are often in a better position to evaluate and prescribe drugs, and their advice should be followed by the consumer, some participants felt.

Participants considered the following options for achieving the benefits for the center while minimizing its risks:

1. Incorporate the center's proposed objectives into existing programs with some form of advisory board to oversee the activities.

2. Establish the proposed center with reliable surveillance and evaluation procedures. Ensure that existing programs maintain current status such as employment and research funding.
3. Proceed with the center in two phases.
   a. Integrate the national center into existing programs (without its own lab and hospital). Begin structuring the activities of the center at a low cost.
   b. After a few years, establish a laboratory and hospital that could then bring in personnel and projects from other areas. This would permit a gradual transition from decentralized and dispersed information and resources to centralization.

6

Recombinant DNA Techniques and New Drugs: Science, Policy, and Ethics

Since life on this planet began about 4 billion years ago, all organisms have carried their hereditary information in a substance called DNA (deoxyribonucleic acid). For billions of years DNA molecules were the preeminent information processing devices on earth. As Carl Sagan has noted, it was not until the Carboniferous Period—about 300 to 350 million years ago—that animal brains grew large enough to surpass the information-processing capacity of the DNA molecule. For the first time in history a creature existed that had more information in its brains than in its genes. Since the Carboniferous Period, much of history can be described as the gradual (and certainly incomplete) dominance of brains over genes.[1]

Every day, the cells of the human body produce a wide array of chemicals which are still beyond production techniques of our current technology. Recombinant DNA techniques allow genetic material of one organism to be transplanted into another, so that the second cell operates in some altered way. This is important both for the production of certain drugs now beyond the capacity of industrial chemistry, such as insulin or the brain hormone somatostatin, and for gene replacement therapy (the use of viruses to carry correcting messages directly to the genes).

This chapter reviews the scientific basis of genetics and recombinant DNA techniques, the recent history of their development and use in making pharmaceuticals and related therapies, the nature of the policy debate, and several additional ethical and policy questions.

[1]Carl Sagan, *The Dragons of Eden: Speculations on the Evolution of Human Intelligence* (New York: Ballantine Books, 1977), p. 49.

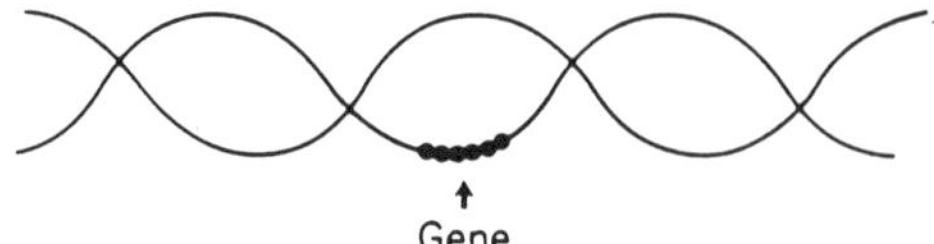

Figure 6-1. Schematic representation of deoxyribonucleic acid (DNA). DNA in each cell contains the genetic information that determines the traits of the organism. The dots on the double-stranded helix designate specific genes. [SOURCE: Used with permission from Herbert Weissbach, "Recombinant DNA—A General Review," Paper Presented at the Symposium on the Social and Ethical Implications of Recent Developments in Science and Technology, 1977 (City University of New York, December 7–9, 1977).]

RECOMBINANT DNA: A GENERAL REVIEW[2]

DNA is the genetic material in all living cells. In higher organisms it is contained in the nucleus of the cell. It carries the genetic information for all inherited characteristics such as eye, skin, and hair color, sex, and metabolic activity. DNA is a long, double-stranded molecule (a "double helix") which, in the cell, is highly coiled and may be circular (see Figure 6-1). Each strand of DNA is composed of four basic chemicals linked together in long chains; these four chemicals are present in the DNA of all cells from the most primitive organisms to human beings. It is in the sequence of these chemicals that the genetic information exists, and it is this information that determines the characteristics of the organism.

The gene is the basic unit of heredity. A gene can be thought of as the smallest piece of DNA that contains the information for a specific trait. Generally, the greater the amount of DNA in a cell, the greater the number of genes present. For example, a single bacterium such as *Escherichia coli* (*E. coli*) may contain 2,000 to 4,000 genes, whereas an animal cell may have more than 50,000 genes. Genes are arranged along chromosomes, which may be pictured as discrete packages containing large numbers of genes. *E. coli* contains 1 or 2 chromosomes, whereas a human cell has 46 chromosomes. Every cell of an organism has the same genetic material: the liver, heart, and skin all have the same DNA, yet the structure and function of individual organs are quite different.

[2]This section is adapted with permission from Herbert Weissbach, "Recombinant DNA—A General Review," Paper Presented at the Symposium on the Social and Ethical Implications of Recent Developments in Science and Technology, 1977 (City University of New York, December 7–9, 1977).

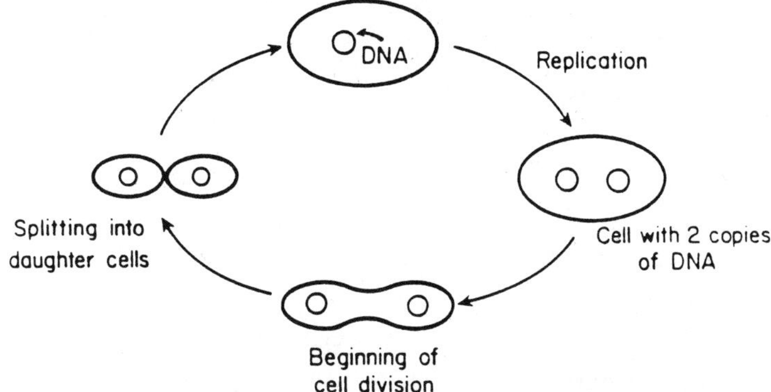

Figure 6-2. Steps involved in bacterial cell division. Replication of DNA precedes the splitting into daughter cells. [Used with permission from same source as Figure 6-1.]

When a cell divides, the daughter cell contains an exact copy of the parent's DNA. In this way, cell division ensures that all the cells of an organism contain the same DNA (see Figure 6-2). When a cell is ready to divide, it duplicates its DNA. When division occurs, each daughter cell receives an exact copy of the DNA. Thus, identical genetic information is passed from cell to cell. If a cell divides rapidly, large numbers of cells and, accordingly, large quantities of DNA may be obtained within a relatively brief period of time. This is crucial to experiments using recombinant DNA techniques.

As mentioned above, each gene contains the genetic information for a specific trait. In biochemical terms, however, it is more accurate to say that each gene contains the information for the structure of one protein. By a complex series of reactions, the cell uses the information in DNA to synthesize proteins from their basic building blocks, amino acids (see Figure 6-3). There are 20 different amino acids. The sequence of the four chemicals that comprise the DNA molecule determines the sequence of amino acids in the proteins. Thus, the proteins

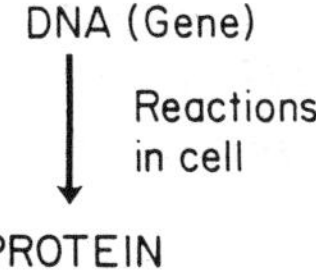

Figure 6-3. Expression of genetic information. Each gene contains the information for a specific protein. [Used with permission from same source as Figure 6-1.]

Table 6-1. Structure and Function of Proteins

A. Structure
   1. Composed of long chains of amino acids linked together. The sequence of amino acids in a protein is determined by the DNA in the cell.

B. Function in cells
   1. Enzymes—to metabolize foods and catalyze chemical reactions in cells
   2. Hormones—insulin, growth hormones, etc.
   3. Structural proteins—skin, muscle
   4. Antibodies—protect cells against foreign substances
   5. Special functions—hemoglobin, rhodopsin, interferon

SOURCE: Used with permission from Herbert Weissbach, "Recombinant DNA—A General Review," Paper Presented at the Symposium on the Social and Ethical Implications of Recent Developments in Science and Technology, 1977 (City University of New York, December 7–9, 1977).

in the cell represent the final expression of genetic information. Proteins have essential functions in many cellular processes: they act as hormones, enzymes, and structural components as well as perform a variety of other special functions (see Table 6-1).

Picture DNA as a computer tape containing information that the cell can retrieve in the form of proteins. Each cell retrieves or expresses the information from the DNA that it needs to function. Thus, the cell is able to regulate the expression of the individual genes in its DNA. This process of regulation is currently one of the most important areas of research, for it relates to a wide variety of physiological conditions.

In order to understand the current concept of gene regulation, it may be helpful to examine a schematic representation of a region on the DNA (see Figure 6-4). The gene has the information that will determine the structure of a specific protein if the gene is expressed. This is referred to as the *structural region.* Adjacent to the structural region is a segment called the *regulatory region*, which regulates whether or not the gene will be expressed. It does not contain information for a specific protein. The regulatory region can be pictured as an on-off switch that responds to biochemical signals. For example, the hormone insulin is produced by specific cells in the pancreas. The regulatory region in these cells is sensitive to changes in blood glucose levels, so that insulin is synthesized according to demand for the hormone. Although the cells of other organs also contain the gene for

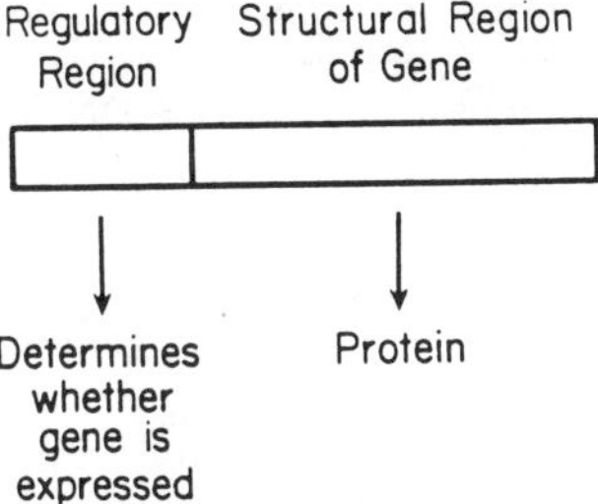

Figure 6-4. Schematic representation of a genetic region showing structural and regulatory regions. [Used with permission from same source as Figure 6-1.]

insulin production, the regulatory region is not activated and no insulin is produced.

An understanding of the regulation of gene expression is fundamental to many areas of biology. The differentiation of tissue that occurs during the development of the embryo, the transformation of a normal cell into a malignant cell, the events that take place after a virus infects a cell, and the nature of genetic diseases are examples of problems involving regulation of gene expression. Sickle cell anemia is a classic example—a defect in the DNA alters the cell's ability to synthesize a particular amino acid in the hemoglobin molecule. Although only 1 amino acid out of more than 100 is abnormal, it alters the ability of the sickle cell hemoglobin to carry oxygen. It is also possible to have a defect in the regulatory region adjacent to the gene. Such a defect could prevent the gene from turning on, so that the protein either is not made or is produced in insufficient quantity.

If large amounts of specific genetic regions could be obtained, the chemical and molecular structure of DNA could be studied, and progress could be made in understanding the regulation of gene expression. This is one reason why the technique of recombinant DNA is so important to scientists in this field.

Recombinant DNA technology permits the movement of segments of DNA from one species to another. During the past 5 years, this process has been refined and simplified so that scientists can readily use the technique in their studies. DNA can be cut into small segments by restriction endonucleases, enzymes (proteins that act as biological catalysts) that cleave the DNA strands at particular points. This is one way of obtaining a short segment of DNA (donor DNA) containing certain genes that can potentially be moved into another organism.

Table 6-2. Terms Used in Recombinant DNA Studies

Term	Definition	Note
Recombinant DNA	technique to recombine DNA (genes) of one species with another	
Restriction endonuclease	enzyme that cuts DNA at specific sites	
Plasmid	nonchromosomal bacterial DNA	Both used as vectors
Bacteriophage	bacterial virus	Both used as vectors
Containment	biological and physical means to minimize potential risk	

SOURCE: Used with permission from same source as Table 6-1.

Currently, most recombinant DNA experiments use *E. coli* K12, a strain of the organism *Escherichia coli*, as the host into which the donor DNA is inserted. *E. coli* K12 is used because it has a short generation time (dividing in 20 to 30 minutes), has been extensively studied, and is known to be harmless to humans.

Plasmids and bacteriophages (see Table 6-2) are used in recombinant DNA experiments as vectors to transmit the donor DNA into host organisms. Both plasmids and bacteriophages contain small DNA molecules that can readily enter the *E. coli* K12 host cell. Plasmids are small, circular nonchromosomal DNA species containing a small number of genes that can enter bacterial cells and replicate like chromosomal DNA. A typical bacteriophage is a virus containing DNA that can infect bacterial cells. In some cases, the infection causes the cell to lyse, or disintegrate. In others, the viral DNA becomes integrated into the host cell DNA and replicates with it. Obviously, if the donor DNA can be attached to the vector DNA, it would be possible to move the donor DNA into the host. Table 6-3 describes

Table 6-3. Containment Gradations for Recombinant DNA Experiments

Biological—weakened strains of *E. coli* K12 (EK1, EK2)
Physical—Special laboratories (P1–P4)

- P1—good laboratory procedures, trained personnel, wastes decontaminated
- P2—biohazards sign, no public access, autoclave in building, hand-washing facility
- P3—negative pressure, filters in vacuum line, class II safety cabinets
- P4—Monolithic construction, air locks, all air decontaminated, autoclave in room, all experiments in class II safety cabinets (glove box), shower room

SOURCE: Used with permission from same source as Table 6-1.

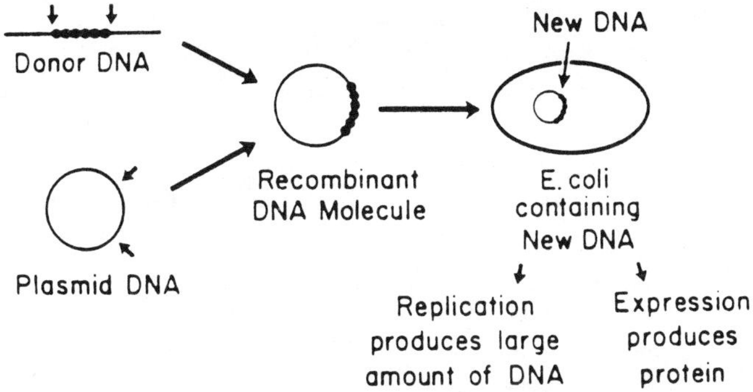

Figure 6-5. Technique of recombinant DNA. The individual steps are described in the text. [Used with permission from same source as Figure 6-1.]

physical and biological containment methods used to minimize potential risk of recombinant DNA experiments.

Plasmids, which are easily isolated from bacteria, can also be cut by restriction enzymes. DNA fragments are "sticky." By simply mixing the donor and plasmid DNA after they have been cut, it is possible to obtain molecules that contain donor DNA loosely associated with plasmid DNA. Special enzymes are then used to seal the DNA pieces together to form a recombinant DNA molecule—a molecule containing DNA from the donor and the plasmid.

The bacterial host, *E. coli* K12, can be treated in such a way that the recombinant DNA plasmid will enter the cell and be present as a nonchromosomal piece of DNA. Two potential reactions can then occur. If the DNA of the organism replicates and the cell divides, it would be possible to obtain large amounts of DNA in a short period of time. This offers a unique way of studying gene regions from higher organisms, especially the regulatory regions. These studies on the fine structure of DNA would undoubtedly lead to important knowledge of gene structure, function, and regulation. In addition, the DNA could be expressed by the host cell. If, for example, the insulin gene was placed into the host cell, its expression would lead to the synthesis of insulin by the cell. The bacterial production of insulin would provide an inexpensive and essentially limitless source of the hormone. In this way, many scarce, important biological products could conceivably be produced. The value of this new technique is apparent. It not only provides a way of obtaining large amounts of DNA for study, but it also provides a novel means for the biological production of proteins.

A simplified schematic representation of a typical experiment is shown in Figure 6-5. At the upper left is the donor DNA containing genes that are to be moved. The arrows designate the regions on the DNA where restriction enzymes cut the molecule into short segments. At the bottom left is a plasmid that will serve as the vector. It should be stressed that there are many variations of the technique depicted in Figure 6-5. Basically, however, all recombinant DNA experiments involve a donor DNA, a vector to move the DNA, and a host to accept the donor DNA.

POTENTIAL APPLICATION OF RECOMBINANT DNA TECHNOLOGY IN PHARMACEUTICAL AND MEDICAL THERAPY

New approaches to genetic research could provide significant future advances in medicine, agriculture, industry, and basic research. Appendix A (page 124) identifies several of these. Most of the recent news about recombinant DNA research in industry has focused on the use of genetic engineering to produce drugs and other chemicals. Scientists have long appreciated the fact that nature can synthesize chemicals that are far too complex for modern technology. Not only is this biological synthesis capable of making more complex macromolecules, but it can do so with much greater efficiency and little or no pollution.[3]

The pharmaceutical industry is seeking to make use of nature's productive elegance and efficiency by using DNA techniques to produce a variety of proteins and other macromolecules such as insulin, somatostatin, and interferon. Insulin, for example, is currently extracted from animal tissue at great cost: enormous amounts of tissue are required to extract minute amounts of the pure hormone. Some patients suffer undesirable allergic reactions to insulin produced in this manner. DNA techniques have been used to produce human insulin by placing the human gene for insulin production into bacteria. Not only might allergic reactions be minimized, but production costs will be lowered significantly. Similarly, where an effective vaccine produces toxic side effects, its constituent virus might be modified so that toxicity is eliminated.

A different approach to therapy through recombinant DNA technology would work to cure underlying defects through gene

[3]James F. Danielli, "Artificial Synthesis of New Life Forms," *Bulletin of the Atomic Scientists* (December, 1972), pp. 20–24.

replacement therapy. Biomedical researchers are exploring methods of reaching directly into the cell to replace incorrect genetic material:

> . . . There are a number of genetic diseases, labeled collectively "inborn errors of metabolism," which result from the absence or severe reduction in the patient of a particular enzyme. Diseases caused in these cases either through the accumulation of the substance which the enzyme is supposed to destroy or convert, or by reducing the availability of the product of the enzyme's reaction.
>
> The deficiency of particular enzymes will be overcome through gene (replacement) therapy. Microbiologists working with viruses that bear the deficient enzyme will literally replace the missing genetic information in a human cell simply by giving the patient a viral infection. The virus will then transmit to the human the genetic information necessary to make the enzyme.[4]

This approach to disease—the alteration of underlying physiological causes of illness—is potentially important in the treatment of diabetes. DNA research may tell scientists why the pancreatic cells of certain diabetics do not produce enough insulin. DNA technology can be used to identify the normal controlling steps in insulin gene activation and may reveal the molecular lesion underlying some types of diabetes.[5] To the extent that cancer has a genetic basis, gene replacement therapy may eventually have applications in cancer treatment.

RECENT DEVELOPMENTS IN THE USE AND REGULATION OF RECOMBINANT DNA

Since 1974 DNA issues have attracted significant attention from both the scientific and the lay press. In addition to frequent coverage in publications such as *Science*, *Nature*, and *Science News*, helpful information can be found in the work of the House Health and Environment Subcommittee and the August, 1978, "Oversight Report of the Senate Commerce Subcommittee on Science Technology and Space." Much of this attention has focused on the possibility of biohazards resulting from the research itself, the guidelines established by NIH

[4]Policy Research Inc., "A Comprehensive Study of the Ethical, Legal, and Social Implications of Advances in Biomedical and Behavioral Research and Technology," Final Report and Summary of Responses to the First Policy Evaluation Instrument (Baltimore, 1977), p. 274.

[5]North Atlantic Assembly, Scientific and Technical Committee, "Draft Information Document on Recombinant DNA" (May, 1978).

Table 6-4. Containment Recommended by the National Institutes of Health for Recombinant DNA Experiments, 1978

Donor DNA	*Host*	*Containment*
Primate (nonembryonic)	*E. coli*	P4 + EK2
Primate (embryonic)	*E. coli*	P3 + EK2
Other mammals	*E. coli*	P3 + EK2
Birds	*E. coli*	P3 + EK2
Cold-blooded animals	*E. coli*	P2 + EK1
Animal virus	*E. coli*	P4 + EK2

SOURCE: Used with permission from same source as Table 6-1.

to ensure safe research, the question of voluntary compliance by industry with the guidelines, and the patentability of processes and products of DNA research.

Scientists and laypersons alike have been concerned about the degree of biohazard associated with DNA research. These concerns were articulated in a letter written by Paul Berg, one of the discoverers of the recombinant DNA technique. Joined by nine other researchers in the field, he called for a voluntary halt to recombinant DNA experiments until guidelines could be developed to ensure the safety of the research.

In response, NIH sponsored a conference in Asilomar, California. Experts in recombinant DNA technology gathered to develop preliminary guidelines for research, which were issued in 1976. The guidelines require both physical and biological containment. Physical containment requirements become more stringent as the degree of possible danger increases. Containment measures are graduated from P1 and P2 levels of minimum isolation, to the P3 level of moderate isolation, to the P4 level of maximum isolation (see Table 6-3). Biological containment refers to the use of host strains of *E. coli* that are genetically crippled so that they cannot survive outside special laboratory conditions. Table 6-4 outlines the type of physical and biological containment required for different types of donor DNA in the earliest NIH guidelines.

Since 1976 a variety of experiments have shown that there is little danger from the research activities when proper control is exercised. The recent meeting of the Committee on Genetic Experimentation of the International Council of Scientific Unions (COGENE) reflected the attitudes of most microbiologists. The group stated, "Most scientists working in the field now believe that the original fears were based on bad scientific judgment, and that recombinant DNA experiments at their very worst can pose no more hazard than that of working with the most dangerous organism involved in the experiment."[6]

Because of the diminished level of risk that has been shown, NIH revised the guidelines in 1979 so that certain kinds of experiments could be done with lower levels of physical and biological containment. Nevertheless, many feel that the guidelines have a major flaw in that they can be enforced only against institutions receiving NIH funding; industry and other privately funded research institutions are not subject to the guidelines.

Part of the recombinant DNA research success story is due to industry involvement. Several large pharmaceutical firms have entered the field including Abbott Laboratories, Eli Lilly, Hoffmann-La Roche, Merck, Sharp & Dohme, Pfizer, and Upjohn. Recognition of the technology's potential has also brought about the establishment of several new companies devoted exclusively to the development of new drugs and other products using recombinant DNA technology. The Cetus Corporation in Berkeley and Genentech in San Francisco are the best known, although three more companies—Biogen in Luxembourg, Genex in Rockville, Maryland, and Bethesda Research Laboratories in Bethesda, Maryland—have been established. These companies have begun active research into the production of substances such as insulin, interferon, vaccines, and food products.[7] The rapid growth of these small companies, representing the efforts of university researchers and financing raised in the venture capital market, has involved more than $150 million.[8]

As noted previously, private companies are currently under no formal restrictions on recombinant DNA research, although they are encouraged to register voluntarily with NIH and to comply with the guidelines. However, only one company had registered as of May, 1979, and at least one is already planning to conduct experiments involving more than 10 liters of culture without receiving formal NIH approval as required by the guidelines. This has made mandatory compliance a serious consideration in Congress and NIH.

Patentability of recombinant DNA processes and products has been

[6]Eleanor Lawrence, "Guidelines Should Go, DNA Meeting Concludes," *Nature*, Vol. 278, No. 5705 (April 12, 1979), p. 590.

[7]David Dickson, "U.S. Drug Companies Push for Changes in Recombinant DNA Guidelines," *Nature*, Vol. 278, No. 5703 (March 29, 1979), pp. 385–386.

[8]David Dickson, "Recombinant DNA Research: Private Actions Raise Public Eyebrows." *Nature*, Vol. 278, No. 5704 (April 5, 1979), pp. 494–495.

a troubling issue. NIH has encouraged companies to apply for a patent before registering work with NIH. Nevertheless, companies have been unwilling to register even completed research projects until judicial or legislative clarification of the patentability of DNA products is assured. At the direction of the U.S. Supreme Court, the Court of Customs and Patent Appeals has reexamined and reaffirmed its decision that patent applications on micro-organisms could be granted to General Electric. In June, 1980, the Supreme Court affirmed the Appeals Court ruling that patents can be granted on genetically engineered micro-organisms.

LONG-TERM ISSUES

As recombinant DNA research continues and its momentum grows, a series of questions arises regarding long-term aspects of this technology. These questions concern the propriety of human control of evolution, the allocation of costs for development of DNA technology, and the long-term social benefits likely to result.

When assessing the social impacts of genetic engineering, many scientists feel that the most important advances from recombinant DNA research will be increased knowledge of the basic elements of life. The scientific community generally agrees that long-term effects, both positive and negative, of broader knowledge have not received as much attention as immediate questions of biohazards. Examples of the potential long-term consequences are contained in a study prepared for the National Commission for the Protection of Human Subjects of Biomedical and Behavioral Research. This study examines some of the issues raised when the focus moves beyond research to application of new therapies.[9] An expert panel examined a variety of technologies including gene replacement therapy. Panelists generally viewed gene replacement therapy with some alarm, particularly with regard to possible long-term consequences of genetic manipulation and difficulties of assessing those consequences.

Scientists have predicted that recombinant DNA technology has great potential for curing certain diseases and correcting genetic errors. The question is whether public funds should be allocated to recombinant DNA research as distinct from research into other ap-

[9] Policy Research Inc., *op. cit.*, pp. 62–73.

proaches to health. The impressive advances in molecular genetics have been attributed to federal support of biomedical research to conquer the "killer diseases" such as cancer and cardiovascular disease.[10] In terms of health outcomes, other approaches to biomedical research—particularly disease prevention and health promotion including the removal of environmental pollutants—may have higher immediate health payoffs for a large number of people. When asked to choose among the most important of several approaches to the extension of life, the expert panel chose control of the environmental causes of disease and trauma by a three-to-one margin over gene replacement therapy.[11]

It is true that benefits might accrue from changing from a palliative to an interventive mode in caring for inborn errors of metabolism. Such an approach might reduce the cost of medical treatment and lead to a new view of "chronic" diseases—those not subject to gene replacement therapy. But if gene replacement therapy is successful in extending life, it is important to consider the social and economic costs that would accompany the increasing age of the population.

The allocation issue is also relevant to the distribution of benefits of recombinant DNA research. While some benefits may indeed go to poor or minority patients, such as black persons suffering from sickle cell anemia, the benefits initially are likely to be administered by major medical centers.

Another important issue concerns the ethics of conscious control of evolution by humans. As it is currently conceived, gene replacement therapy might alter the gene pool. Successful use of such therapy to repair defects in metabolism might lead to demands for use of the technology in enhancing human function. Concerns of molecular biologists over biohazards has not generated broad public discussion of long-term impacts such as control of evolution. That debate exists, but it has not been elevated to the level that accompanied the threat of the release of toxic and resistant new life forms. Some observers have compared recombinant DNA technology to nuclear power and urged molecular biologists to focus public scrutiny on the long-term effects of their work. Significant questions relating to these long-term effects of recombinant DNA technology include:[12]

[10]Clifford Grobstein, "The Recombinant-DNA Debate," *Scientific American* (July, 1977), pp. 22–23.

[11]Policy Research Inc., *op. cit.*, p. 84.

[12]"Molecular Biology: Suffering from Shock," *Nature*, Vol. 278, No. 5705 (April 12, 1979), p. 587.

- Do humans have the right to change their genetic nature? Would changing the genetic structure affect the sense of self and notions about the meaning of life?
- What effect would it have on the gene pool?
- Should persons who have undergone gene replacement therapy procreate? Would their procreation pass on unknown changes to the next generation?
- If effective gene replacement were available, would it be required of those receiving public support to ameliorate conditions that could be cured? For example, could welfare benefits be denied to sickle cell anemia victims who refused to undergo gene replacement therapy?
- Could gene replacement lead to the development of a "superior" class?
- What side effects are possible? For example, could cancer or autoimmune reactions result?

APPENDIX A

Applications of Recombinant DNA Technology

The ability to manipulate genetic information has a wide range of applications in addition to drug development. The Congressional Office of Technology Assessment has compiled the following preliminary list of potential applications for genetic research:

Primary food production
- Grains
- Vegetables
- Fruits

Livestock production
- Improving current stocks

Nonfood plants and animals
- Ornamental plants
- Pets

Materials production
- Wood
- Fibers

Food fermentation products
- Beverages
- Cheeses
- Other foods

Pharmaceutical products
- Antibiotics
- Antibodies
- Vaccines
- Enzymes
- Hormones
- Psychoactive agents/stimulants, depressants, relaxants

Scavengers of pollutants

Concentrators of scarce materials

Products from biomass
- Energy (methane, ammonia)
- Ammonia
- Fertilizers
- Chemical feedstocks

Manufactured foods

HIGHLIGHTS OF THE DISCUSSION

Due to the many unknowns relating to DNA technology, there was a great deal of disagreement over the problems of regulation, ethics, control of human evolution, and effects on lifespan.

Herbert Weissbach, associate director of the Roche Institute of Molecular Biology, outlined the science of DNA, including the chemical components of DNA (A, C, G, and T), the cell division process, the regulation of gene expression, recombinant DNA techniques, and research (see pages 112–118). Burke Zimmerman, director of the NIH Division of Legislative Analysis and formerly a staff member of the Health and Environment Subcommittee of the House Interstate and Foreign Commerce Committee, reviewed the history of government regulation of DNA.

Early NIH guidelines were begun in 1974 and were formally released on June 23, 1976, he explained. There was concern regarding private sector research that was not necessarily under government jurisdiction. Congressional action began to consider extending guidelines to that sector. The debate became heated and led to proposals for stringent regulations, but as the debate subsided, so did support for more severe measures.

At the end of 1978 there was again an effort at passing legislation. The new effort raised the question of where the government has authority to regulate. Currently, the NIH guidelines include voluntary compliance. Drug industry spokespeople seem to feel that the guidelines are a good idea, provide for a great deal of flexibility, and are reasonable in that exemptions are possible. Some company leaders, however, say that if guidelines are too restrictive, companies will move on their own to circumvent them. Currently, there is disagreement among the different groups—research, government, and industry—over whether voluntary federal regulation is sufficient and what the future will bring. In 1980, the guidelines were made less stringent, although they continue to be applied to industry on a voluntary basis.

Leroy Walters, director of the Center for Bioethics of Georgetown University's Kennedy Institute of Ethics, gave an example of speculative ethics. He outlined the ethical issues that would be raised with the first use of recombinant DNA technique of gene replacement therapy for single gene defects such as sickle cell anemia.

1. Research design: The aim of research should be to maximize information and minimize risk to the subject. Therefore, a risk-benefit analysis is crucial. Difficulties include the fact that few animal models exist for single gene defects and the question of whether very serious diseases justify more dangerous risks.
2. Equitable selection of subjects: If certain racial or ethnic groups suffer a disease, does the use of gene replacement therapy for them imply that they are "expendable people" on whom researchers can perform their first experiments?
3. Informed consent: The quality of disclosure to volunteers is important because DNA research is a new area in medicine and the risks and benefits are still unknown. Research subjects should be aware of this fact.
4. Injury: Compensation for injured subjects should be available. Researchers and society should feel a moral obligation to compensate subjects for injury, since the experiments are for the good of society.
5. Allocation of resources: Would the funds used in gene replacement therapy be better spent in treating or preventing other diseases?
6. The line between therapy and genetic engineering and the related concepts of health and disease: Is there a threshold condition for using gene replacement therapy? For example, lethargy and exhaustion are two of the symptoms of sickle cell anemia; how much lethargy and exhaustion make the disease serious enough to use gene replacement?

In the discussion that followed the presentations, it was noted that no existing regulatory board has among its members the full range of scientific, medical, engineering, and economic expertise necessary to judge DNA research in advance. We do not know what a "good" experiment is until it is done.

There are also risks of scale in experiments. The question arises as to how to protect society given the larger amounts of the substance that are needed for research. Guidelines should outline reasonable levels of containment. In most research this is not a problem because the amounts in current use are small, but in the manufacture of chemicals (e.g., insulin) large amounts would be necessary.

The question of whether recombinant DNA gives us more conscious control of human evolution than humans have ever had led to consideration of the ethical and policy implications of this potential control. One research scientist argued that certain drugs, particularly penicillin, had a greater effect on human evolution (by allowing large numbers of people who would have died of infectious and other diseases to live long enough to reproduce) than gene replacement therapy will ever have. Besides, according to this line of argument, recombinant DNA is still in an early stage, and it is too early to know what the ethical issues really are. Raising them now, in the absence of facts, could lead to premature regulation.

There was disagreement over when it will be possible to control genetic trials. Some participants argued that the uncertainty of DNA research is all the greater reason to raise ethical issues now. This is the approach taken by the Office of Technology Assessment (OTA), which is currently examining the issues surrounding nonhuman (plants, animals, and single cell) applications of DNA technologies on the assumption that it will take a long time to prepare for policy decisions and that the potential impacts should be explored now.

It was suggested that perhaps a different type of decision process is needed, possibly one that includes methods of developing widespread public consensus on these issues. Some participants criticized the notion that all members of the public, particularly the uneducated, could not contribute to this decision process. Participants from the OTA replied that their experience and that of other researchers has shown that average citizens can identify impacts and make interpretations not seen by researchers. Also, there are decisionmaking techniques that allow officials and citizens to explore technological options in relation to their values.

There was also disagreement over whether those people now alive would live longer because of recombinant DNA techniques. The possibility of significant changes in society because of altered age cohorts raised the question of whether research funds should be allocated to prolong life or to ensure adequate resources for those who are elderly.

Speakers at the Foresight Seminars on Pharmaceutical R & D

"THE FUTURE OF PHARMACEUTICALS: BREAKTHROUGH POSSIBILITIES, DEVELOPMENT CONSTRAINTS, AND POLICY QUESTIONS"

Jerome E. Schnee, Ph.D., Associate Professor, Graduate School of Business, Rutgers University, a leading writer on industrial innovation particularly in the pharmaceutical area, who has given particular attention to the interaction of government regulation and innovation.

Frank G. Standaert, M.D., Chairman, Department of Pharmacology, School of Medicine, Georgetown University, a member of the National Research Council and of the editorial boards of major pharmacology journals in the United States, author of more than 70 articles and reports in the field of pharmacology.

James Turner, J.D., of Swankin & Turner, a public interest law firm, author of *Chemical Feast: The Nader Report on the Food and Drug Administration*, a frequent consultant to various congressional committees and consumer groups on food and drug issues.

"THE RISE OF ALTERNATIVES TO DRUG THERAPIES AND THE IMPLICATIONS FOR PHARMACEUTICAL R & D"

Rick J. Carlson, J.D., Senior Associate, Commonweal Research Institute, and President of Health Resources and Communications Inc., a frequent consultant to the Department of Health, Education, and Welfare and to House and Senate committees on health issues, author of *The End of Medicine*, a major review of the health care system and a precursor of the holistic health movement.

Shelia Touquan, R.Ph., M.S., J.D., National Drug Program Coordinator, Blue Cross and Blue Shield Associations, a registered pharmacist and an expert on pharmaceutical policy, particularly reimbursement issues, who directs one of the largest drug reimbursement programs in the country.

Murray Weiner, M.D., Vice President for Research and Scientific Affairs of the Merrell Research Center, a clinical pharmacologist and hematologist, author of over 180 scientific papers, a book on coagulation, and *The Medicine Makers*, a novel about medical research.

"THE IMPACT OF REGULATION ON INCENTIVES FOR PHARMACEUTICAL R & D"

William S. Comanor, Ph.D., Director of the Bureau of Economics of the Federal Trade Commission, Professor of Economics, University of California at Santa Barbara, and a leading student of industrial innovation and advertising with extensive teaching experience, who has frequently advised congressional committees and served as Special Economic Assistant to the head of the Antitrust Division of the Justice Department.

Leon I. Goldberg, Ph.D., M.D., Professor of Pharmacology and Medicine and Director of Clinical Pharmacology at the University of Chicago, a clinical pharmacologist who has discovered and tested new drug therapies, particularly for treating shock, who serves on a variety of academic and governmental review panels, and has published widely on clinical research methods and drug therapies.

Hubert C. Peltier, M.D., Senior Vice President for Development of the Merck, Sharp and Dohme Research Laboratories, an industry researcher and executive with experience in a variety of companies, who is a frequent participant in government panels, including the Adverse Drug Reaction Panel of the Office of Technology Assessment.

"THE IMPACT OF NATIONAL HEALTH INSURANCE ON PHARMACEUTICAL R & D"

Peter Goldschmidt, M.D., Dr. P.H., D.M.S., Vice President of Policy Research Incorporated, author of several major studies of biomedical research, health care evaluation, medical manpower, and medical information systems, who has also designed assessments of the impact of National Health Insurance.

Michael Riddiough, Pharm.D., M.P.H., Senior Analyst in the Health Program of the Office of Technology Assessment, a clinical pharmacist and expert in health policy from the University of California at San Francisco, in charge of OTA's pharmaceutical-related research.

John Virts, Ph.D., Corporate Economist with Eli Lilly & Co. and a leading industry economist, whose specialties include trends in pharmaceutical marketing and sales as well as decision-making factors in pharmaceutical R & D investment.

"THE NATIONAL CENTER FOR DRUG SCIENCE: POLICY QUESTIONS AND LONG-TERM CONSEQUENCES"

John Burns, Ph.D., Vice President—Research of Hoffmann-La Roche Inc., a pharmacologist with extensive government, academic, and industry experience, past president of the American Society of Pharmacology and Experimental Therapeutics, and a member of the National Academy of Sciences and the Institute of Medicine.

Marcia Greenberger, J.D., Director of the Women's Rights Project of the Center for Law and Social Policy, a leading advocate for consumer, civil rights, and women's groups on food and drug issues, a member of the Joint Commission on Prescription Drug Use, and a consultant to the General Accounting Office on evaluations of drug regulation.

John Oates, M.D., Professor of Medicine and Pharmacology and Director of Clinical Pharmacology at Vanderbilt University School of Medicine, a widely published researcher and medical educator, who has served on numerous advisory groups, including the advisory panel for OTA's study of drug bioequivalence and the Pharmacology-Toxicology Review Committee of the National Institute of General Medical Sciences.

"RECOMBINANT DNA AND NEW DRUGS: SCIENCE, POLICY, AND ETHICS"

Leroy Walters, Ph.D., Director of the Georgetown University Center for Bioethics of the Kennedy Institute of Ethics, a leading scholar on ethical issues in the life sciences and a member of the Recombinant DNA Advisory Committee of the National Institutes of Health.

Herbert Weissbach, Ph.D., Associate Director of the Roche Institute of Molecular Biology and Head of the Department of Biochemistry, a specialist in the field of protein synthesis with an interest in the use of newer technologies in molecular biology in the biomedical field, who was a leading researcher at the Laboratory of Clinical Biochemistry of the National Institutes of Health.

Burke Zimmerman, Ph.D., Director of the Division of Legislative Analysis of the National Institutes of Health, a biophysicist with extensive academic experience and work with environmental advocates, who was the Science Advisor to Congressman Paul Rodgers and the House Health and Environment Subcommittee on biomedical research issues.

About the Author

Clement Bezold is a political scientist and futurist. After undergraduate training in international affairs at the Georgetown University School of Foreign Service, he received an M.A. in comparative government and a Ph.D. in American government from the University of Florida. He did research on accountability, participation, and foresight as Assistant Director of the Center for Governmental Responsibility at the University of Florida Law School before founding, with Alvin Toffler, the Institute for Alternative Futures in 1977, with support from Antioch University. A frequent lecturer and adviser on foresight and participation to state legislatures and local governments, he is the editor of *Anticipatory Democracy: People in the Politics of the Future* and co-editor (with James Dator) of *Judging the Future: Alternative Futures for the Legal System.* He is preparing a volume on alternative futures for the U.S. health care system, including pharmaceutical therapies.

About the Institute for Alternative Futures

The Institute for Alternative Futures (1624 Crescent Place, N.W., Washington, D.C. 20009) is a nonprofit, tax-exempt organization whose purpose is to encourage more systematic consideration of the future in policymaking and more effective public participation in the decisions that shape the future. An outgrowth of the work of Alvin Toffler and the Committee on Anticipatory Democracy, the principal areas of the institute's research and technical assistance include anticipatory democracy (citizen goal setting and futures planning for city and state government); legislative foresight (techniques that help legislators, committees, and staff consider emerging issues and the long-term impacts of decisions); and organizational planning (the use of long-term futures planning in organizations, particularly voluntary and public interest organizations). The Institute's current projects focus on the future of the legal system, the health care system, environments for children, and technological innovation.

Index

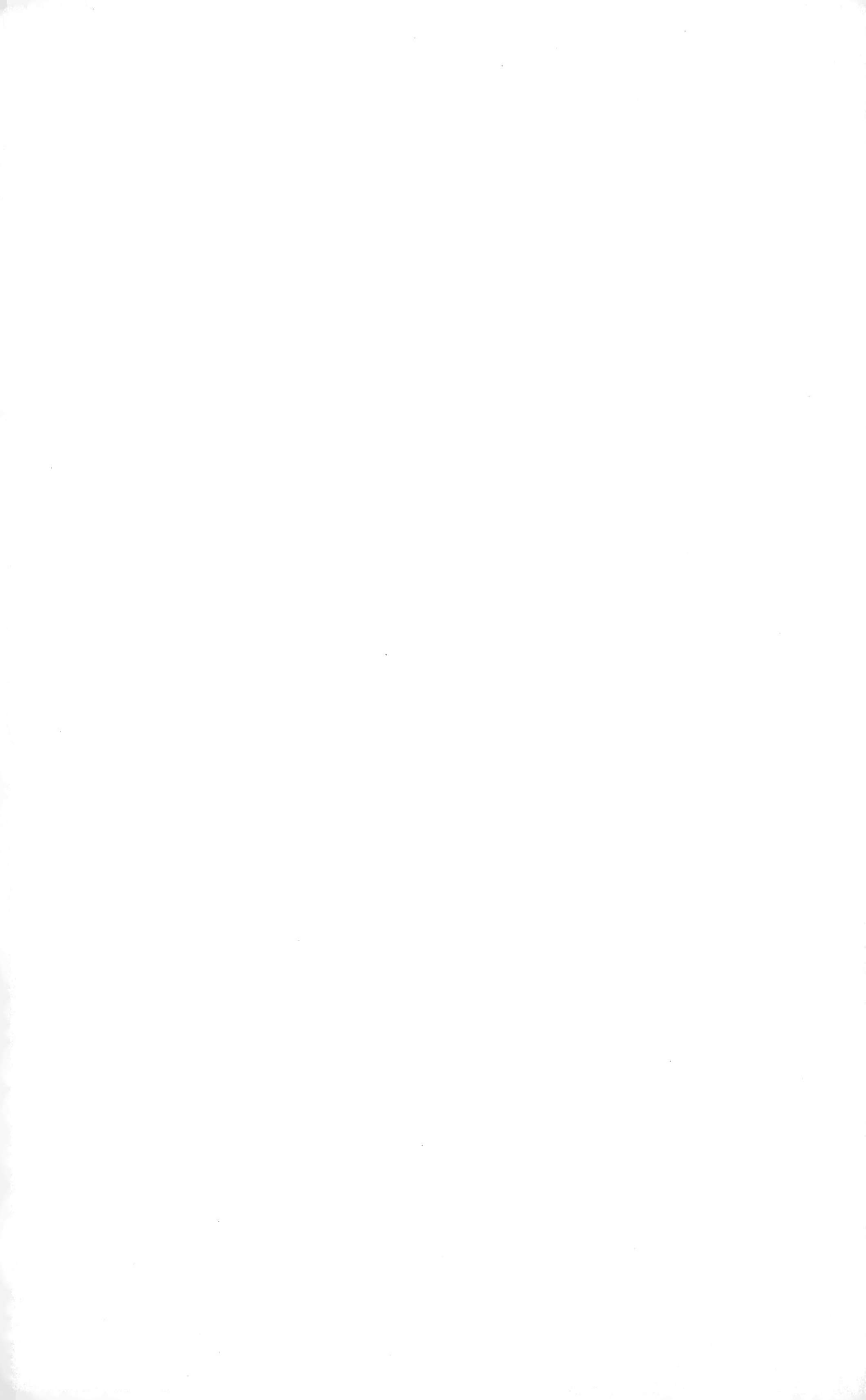